PSYCHIATRY - THEORY, APPLICATIONS AND TREATMENTS

PSYCHOTHERAPY

METHODS, OUTCOMES AND FUTURE DIRECTIONS

PSYCHIATRY - THEORY, APPLICATIONS AND TREATMENTS

Additional books in this series can be found on Nova's website under the Series tab.

Additional e-books in this series can be found on Nova's website under the eBooks tab.

PSYCHIATRY - THEORY, APPLICATIONS AND TREATMENTS

PSYCHOTHERAPY

METHODS, OUTCOMES AND FUTURE DIRECTIONS

DOMINIC BREWER
EDITOR

nova publishers
New York

NOTICE TO THE READER

Library of Congress Cataloging-in-Publication Data

Library of Congress Control Number: 2016938503

ISBN: 978-1-63485-226-5

Published by Nova Science Publishers, Inc. † New York

CONTENTS

PREFACE

This book discusses methods, outcomes and future directions in psychotherapy. Chapter One studies phenomenological hermeneutics psychotherapy. Chapter Two provides an essential understanding of sexual issues so therapists can confidently address problems with both knowledge and strategies that help individuals and/or couples overcome sexual difficulties. Chapter Three explores the emotional needs of people with intellectual disabilities, looking at methods for identifying the issues and ways of working to enable progress to be made. Chapter Four explores the experience of the future because without a sense of the future, patients cannot move forward psychologically.

The remaining chapters are dedicated to the work of Habib Davanloo, MD, Professor Emeritus of Psychiatry at McGill University. The authors in this special section are all current or recent past members of Davanloo's Closed-Circuit Experiential Training Workshops in Major Mobilization of the Unconscious and ISTDP, and have presented at one or more of the last several of Davanloo's annual audio-visual symposia on the metapsychology of the unconscious. All four authors acknowledge a deep sense of gratitude to Dr. Davanloo for his generous sharing of his discoveries and insights, and his tireless teaching. The theoretical concepts presented in these chapters including the terminology such as Mobilization of the Unconscious, Transference Component of the Resistance, Complex Transference Feeling, Unconscious Therapeutic Alliance, Central Dynamic Sequence, Perpetrator of the Unconscious, Fusion of Primitive Murderous Rage with Guilt and Sexuality, Intergenerational Destructive Competitive Transference Neurosis, Uplifting the Transference Neurosis, Unlocking the Unconscious, and others, are not the authors' own. They were developed by Dr. Davanloo by over 50 years of systematic clinical research. Each author, through their many years of involvement in Davanloo's programs brings their own unique synthesis of his teaching. The chapters will review the historical development of Davanloo's ideas and techniques and then will focus on his recent work in Transference Neurosis. The Experiential Training Workshops have provided a laboratory for Dr. Davanloo and the Trainees to get a unique perspective on the Metapsychology of the Unconscious, Unconscious Resistance, Fusion and the various forms of Transference Neurosis. These topics will be elucidated further. It is the hope of the authors, that by the end of this special section, the reader will have a broader understanding of Davanloo's Metapsychology of the Unconscious and of the concept of Transference Neurosis. Further, they hope that their offerings will be useful to psychotherapist of any orientation, to short-term dynamic psychotherapists, and to Davanloo's Intensive Short-Term Dynamic Psychotherapy (DISTDP) therapists specifically as it applies to their most challenging cases.

PART I - RESEARCH ARTICLES

In: Psychotherapy
Editor: Dominic Brewer

ISBN: 978-1-63485-226-5

Chapter 1

PHENOMENOLOGICAL HERMENEUTICS PSYCHOTHERAPY: UNDERSTANDINGS OF HEALTH, ILLNESS AND ETHICS IN CONTEMPORARY

Danielle de Gois Santos*
Universidade Federal do Rio Grande do Norte, Natal, Rio Grande do Norte, Brazil

ABSTRACT

This abstract is based on the thought of the philosopher Martin Heidegger in some of his works, especially Zollikon Seminars. Exercise comprehensive constructed from the literature review is based on hermeneutic-phenomenological method. The proposal essay forewords and a different look on the critical clinical psychology and the processes of disease and promotion of health, paying attention to how they present themselves in the contemporary. Discussions on clinical man-ways to be healthy and be patient and how to be ethical, are made with reference to the experiences of everyday life of the Heideggerian understanding. The work are developed in dialogic relationship with the partnership of other authors such as Hans-Georg Gadamer (1998, 2007, 2011), Michel Foucault (2010), Jeff Malpas (2012), Steven Crowell (2012), etc. Our journey begins with introductory propositions regarding the

* Corresponding author: Danielle de Gois Santos. E-mail: danielledegoissantos@gmail.com.

methodological understanding of hermeneutic phenomenology. Following the work: Health and illness in natural-scientific perspective, Contributions to an understanding of the phenomenology of illness and health care and Ethics in clinical psychology. In this final, if discuss the proposed ethical thinking as a way of being that enables other understandings relating to the subject of existence. The issue of ethics was not taken as a discussion about standards of behavior, but as a reflective exercise/meditation care and freedom, in the ontological sense, implies a transformation of look, reversing the concerns techniques within clinical psychology, exercise ways of being ethical, expanding the possibilities of existential uniqueness.

Keywords: phenomenological hermeneutics, psychotherapy, health, illness, ethics

INTRODUCTION

The natural perspective is prevalent among scientific-research psychological. This chapter sets out to discuss a specific area of psychology, the psychotherapy. In particular, the proposal is to deepen the studies on psychotherapy adopting as toward hermeneutic phenomenological perspective led by philosopher Martin Heidegger.

We are living in increasingly involved simultaneously from different perspectives of reasoning and acting to psychotherapy. Especially the rhythms of life, the professions, the ways in which we are daily asked to live with each other are mediated by quick actions and rare episodes of reflection.

Psychotherapy phenomenological hermeneutic foundation is an invitation for patient and therapist engage in comprehension exercises, reflection and meditation.

The theme of this chapter elucidates about health, illness and ethics in order to invite readers to understand these issues from another look at health, disease and ethics where the former are not opposed and the latter is not a guide of what should and should not do.

Initially, in the first session, Health and Illness are not exclusive of natural-scientific perspectives, reflections will be presented on the dominance that the natural-scientific training influences how we became object health and disease. In turn, the second session, Contributions to a phenomenological understanding of disease, health and ethics, are exposed reflective exercises to understand the phenomena mentioned in psychological practice and our everyday experiences.

METHODS

The research that allows this chapter to born it is foundation bibliographical research. The method which foundation the research and the chapter it is an inheritance of philosophy, hermeneutics. There are many ways to practice Hermeneutics, including associated with various methodologies to be between philosophies and the modern sciences. This time the hermeneutic phenomenology is associated with enabling an exercise understanding of the phenomena, especially the themes of health research, disease and ethics.

HEALTH AND DISEASE ARE NOT EXCLUSIVE OF NATURAL-SCIENTIFIC PERSPECTIVES

Martin Heidegger, German philosopher, brought in his famous work, *Being and Time* (2012) a concern forgotten by science born in modernity, the question the question of the meaning of being. The philosopher innovated to present in his books and conferences the question of the meaning of being so directly linked to daily life to all men.

Health and sickness, in the natural-scientific perspective, are concepts. The contributions of Heidegger to discuss health and disease in psychotherapy phenomenological hermeneutic emphasis on open space to begin to be understood as processes, that not as absolute truths or universal definitions.

Heidegger (2009) questioned the metaphysical foundation of modern science, as understood that this foundation contributed to health and illness are understood as objects. The way the participants of the *Zollikon Seminars*, Heidegger (2009) worked the issues of being causes continually questions about the scientific way of thinking man. For the German philosopher, metaphysical influences to the sciences remember the existence of an absolute knowledge of being, as it were possible to universalize it.

Phenomenology distinguishes the being-there as a being in the world, that is, a being whose essential way is to dwell world, cultivating and caring. Heidegger (2012) as comment in paragraph 42 of *Being and Time*, the being-there is open, as it cultivates the world it inhabits; is constitutively host and openness; is healing; is taken care of; It is taken care of you, with the world and with others.

This understanding helps us to think about the unfeasibility of our efforts on finding causal explanations and objective descriptions of how the man lives and is taken care of. The man, for this study, is one that comes in different ways of being together is the one who can be questioned about his being because it is essentially mere power-be.

The being-there already launched are located in the world, so it is with others, with himself and the world; being-there exists other. For Heidegger (1999), there is no subjectivity or objectivity because there is no split between man and world.

Reflect on ways of illness and health, psychotherapeutic practices and human ethics demand an understanding about the human existence. Welcoming the psic1ologia is not restricted to studying behavior and discourse that transforms men into objects, move seeking to understand the ways of life. This exercise which highlights the fundamental constituents of existence. The questions of existence, highlighted, brought by the Heidegger, paths that allow betting on other possibilities of thinking human.

The phenomena's health and disease do not have the obligation to fit in good or bad values. Health and illness are not necessarily relevant states, only in hospital settings, death, longing for the wellbeing full, etc.

Heidegger (1999, 2009) and the philosopher Hans-Georg Gadamer (2011) help us to think about health and disease through different ways of understanding these phenomena. In this session, both contribute to discuss the influences of the ontological difference, the objectivations and hermeneutics as possible understandings about the concepts of health and disease.

A hermeneutic phenomenological exercise example of inspiration for health debates and disease can be found in Heidegger and Gadamer. Heidegger (2009, 2012) and Gadamer (2011) share the importance given to the issue of "ontological difference," developed by Heidegger (2009). Think of the ontological difference leads to the differentiation between being and being. Heidegger's ontological difference resonates to think ourselves, distinguishing humans from ontic and ontological dimensions.

Heidegger's ontological difference presented by Gadamer (2007), in work *Hermeneutics in Retrospective*, is not taken following the natural-scientific perspective. After explanations of Heidegger (2009) on this subject, what was meant by ontological difference acquires a unique way of thinking being. Thus, according to Gadamer (2007), Heidegger is to be distinguished as "the whole thing," in the tradition.

The hermeneutical exercise was appointed, in Heidegger's thinking, as a break from the influences of German idealism. This session is characterized in our working method to support and develop psychological psychotherapeutic practices. In this sense, we redeemed the late twentieth century, Heidegger experienced the overvaluation of methodological schemes at the expense of attention to the experiences. Thus, the hermeneutical exercise contributes, inspiring today, questioning the devaluation that the phenomena against the growth of objectivations.

Contributions to a Phenomenological Understanding of Health, Disease and Ethics

As the title states, this section, we discuss the contributions to a phenomenological understanding of the suggested themes for the chapter. This means that topics are presented so far to that conventionally they are presented, so do not formulate concepts and theories.

Phenomenological understandings do not hold the phenomena as certain objects. At issue are glimpsed grounds for thinking man's way that contradicts the ways to reduce human beings moved by the free will or the victim.

The Heideggerian works *Being and Time* (2012) and *Zollikon Seminars* (2009) are highlighted by the possibilities in relation to the question of being and the human. These issues contribute to think the themes health and disease, featuring ontological correspondences man-world.

In the works of Heidegger's assertions as to what is fundamentally human existence naming it *Dasein*, *being-there*, being in the world. The existence in phenomenological-hermeneutic perspective, is what the philosopher called opening the clearing. Heidegger (2009) discusses with the participants of the seminars that by experiencing an understanding of the essential foundation of the human being, we need to support the under-the-opening-of-world perception which is veiled. The reflection of Heidegger imposes on the man face his condition of being finite.

Thus, from the influence of Heideggerian reflections, we can establish a comparative, in which man is always relative, and not determined the behavior. Man exists for the condition of being-being. For Heidegger, man, "is 'only' something that is, a being among thousands of other ones and thus dependent, and its being-being, kept incessantly by appropriative event

[*Ereignis*] of being, the unconcealment [*Entbergung*]" (Heidegger, 2009, p. 17). In presenting the mode of existence, this is open and clear.

It is important to clarify that this rationale, anyway there is one way of deprivation. However, in the mode of being sick is even more limited. Usually, the idea that the patient is not the sound accompanies the human way to understand and perform, e.g., healthy.

Every time we admit disease as a state of deprivation, we forget that in modern science, for example, psychiatry and psychology, are linked to the emergence and dominance of illnesses. For Gadamer, "it is, as it were, a subjugation of nature, there where the disease manifests itself. The important thing is to master the disease" (Gadamer, 2011, p. 111). The idea of domination, this science that deal with health, overlooks the possibility that, through the experience of illness, understand how to give our ways of relating and the sense that the sick get in our daily lives.

The illness is referred to as a function that has been changed, close to a nuisance. The sick relates to the restriction of routine, goals and expectations that are part of everyday life. So, how to be ill shown highlighted, while the mode of being healthy is characterized as hidden, without emphasis.

From Heidegger's hermeneutic phenomenology, we can think about health and illness as existential opening modes. The illness is currently showing as a way to think about health. The delimitation of how is our existential gap can not be measured. In practice, we understand the relationships between phenomena and experiences, not an understanding of health and disease object.

Malpas (2012) in the chapter *The collapse of ethical*, causes, "where we are with regard to the reality of ethical practice and ethical commitment?" (Malpas and Crowell, 2012, p. 9). More than highlight an ethical discourse, committed to the senses invested in human-world correspondence, born in the psychotherapeutic joints, a concern with ethics in order to think about issues such as health and disease in the men's daily lives.

To introduce the topic of ethics in the discussions that readers are invited to participate, the proposicion to talk about the ethical codes of the professions. Codes of ethics work, often similar to disciplinary tools. Apparently, we live involved in efforts to reconcile an ethical commitment to prevent us to counter social rules. This assertion is familiar, because in societies worldwide grow disparities, reconciling the character of liberal dynamism and protests to combat growing inequality of rights and duties.

Worldwide, individualities are the kinds of desirable human relationships, as shown in Foucault (2010) in his writings. The capitalist regimes are examples of centralization in individuals, giving the man his experiences positioner. The capitalist regimes often suggest the "isolation" of man: isolated individuals opposing individuals with respect. Thus, we understand that once isolated the human distances herself from his constitutive character relationship and approach devices and practices of control and domination.

A highlight in situations where privilege modes to be individualized, not to say that there was the annihilation of ethics. Isolation of the situations do not fail to highlight the constitutive ethics of human, where we can find ethical commitments. This is because, when isolated, among men grow the ethical difficulties in maintaining commitments.

In phenomenological-hermeneutic perspective, questions about the individualization involve ethics, comprehensive exercises and humanity. In our society, individualized relationships exemplify the ability to reflect on the ethical collapse through separation between man and his relations. Capitalist societies help in the years to reflect on the ethical collapse involving individualism.

When the man is subordinate to the modern technique, approaches what Foucault (2010), in *Hermeneutics of the subject*, discussed the ethics. The man described by the French philosopher is surrounded by historical determination and the ethical dimension. When discussing our practices, Foucault (2010) defends our practices as practices of existence, which reveals a change compared to how human practices are seen as universal or forms of domination.

The way of thinking of Foucault is not isolated, Malpas and Crowell (2012), when referring to the ethical, defend the distant ethics in a practical means of domination or control.

Thematization of Ethics for psychotherapeutic proposal involves the diffusion and call for ethical exercises. These extend into our daily lives, is not just a theoretical question, but heed requests to inhabit the world aiming not just me, but one we.

The crisis accompanying the sciences, in the early twenty-first century, requiring greater justification is the same as that strives in eliminating illnesses, ailments or experiences that somehow demonstrate imbalance. Currently, the scientific field dwells contexts aimed to explain our experiences, from methods that separate man and world. Among the modern sciences, psychology is involved in methods and techniques, as well as lost in the midst of comprehensive exercises, explanatory and requests for specialties which intend to offer resolutions.

For Psychology, as well as other sciences, the metaphysical influences, refer to universal resolutions. The natural resilience movements to achieve universal limited, more and more attention to our everyday how inhabit the world. The science involved in the task of achieving explanations, to the extent that enable its professionals to build understandings about us, our relationships and the world, restricted horizons of possibilities as to how being in the world.

Before scientifically of wanting results, representations, definitions are no made necessary in phenomenological-hermeneutic perspective, questions, admitting that our experiences are always at play in human form. In the scientific system, for example, the requirement to achieve goals does not guarantee that ways of being can be regulated, objectified.

The Exist not if showing a condition capable of being selected or not, but constantly in a dynamic game. Achieving goals or propose objectification does not constitute, for the sciences, necessarily, regulation of lifestyles. Often, illnesses, ways of restricting conditions to be, are devalued and seen as opportunity for regulatory tools are created.

Activities with analysis, diagnosis or descriptions, most of the time, highlight the causes and not the senses involved, for example, phenomena such as health and illness. When investigated, the symptoms of illness in a patient not necessarily consistent with the way they are interpreted. That's because there is a difference between investigating in order to find the cause of illness, and how the phenomenon affects the patient's life. There is a difference between proposed explanations for the experienced illnesses and the ways in which patients experience them.

According to Gadamer (2011), amid artificial ways of thinking about the world and man are open legitimate spaces for formulating knowledge. For the philosopher, the scientific field is legitimated in terms such as "era of positive science." At this stage, metaphysics takes on a new guise. Therefore, science is legitimized holding "realities" and "objects."

The way to experience relationships through hermeneutic exercises, elucidates the design condition, which was proposed by Heidegger, in which men are inserted experiencing the everyday experiences in an unprecedented way. In the design condition, Heidegger's ontological difference leads to critical questioning of our ways of being in the world. The ontological difference contributes to those interested in the reflective exercise are sensitive to issues such as scientific knowledge enhancement.

While working through the exercises to understand and to question during psychotherapy experience are found opportunities for analysis, everyday understandings. So psychotherapeutic experiences are not limited to how questions are valid any prior determinations linked to our experiences. The psychological clinical exercise opportunity presents itself as an opportunity to diversify felt in everyday experiences.

The hermeneutical exercise of everyday relationships enable the possibility to ponder the power of being, Heidegger's existential, our experiences. The existential can be is appropriate in our discussions to understand the usual experiences as inconclusive projects. In everyday life, the existential Heidegger contribute to the rescue of questioning b Gadamer (1998), in *Truth and Method book: basic features of a philosophical hermeneutics*, hermeneutics stands in a direct relationship to understand, referring to hermeneutics as a joint exercise to any man. The hermeneutic thinking, and inspire understandings of the above themes, expresses an understanding of phenomenon that concerns not only the procedures used in the sciences. The scope of hermeneutic thinking beyond ways of conceiving science and goes beyond the scientific and theoretical fields.

The hermeneutical exercise is not restricted exclusively to the skills of modern science. Understanding the exercise presents senses for the experiences and, in due course, reveals the ways in which man relates in the world.

The hermeneutic understanding not only in Gadamer, but mainly in Heidegger, encourages a differentiated and critical look at the psychological clinic. In this clinic, the man is not the center of relations mediated by a universal moral, which regulates the ways of relating. On the contrary, the exercise brings us closer to understanding how to be responsible, to be present in an ethical manner. Thus, the phenomena exhibited at the clinic, once a way of being ethical, from hermeneutic exercises, enables theming instead of particularization (objectification) of the experiences.

Commonly, the modern sciences are accompanied by the presence of interpretive and explanatory speeches prioritized in their applicative capabilities. However, when dealing with interpretive formulations we are referring collectively to understanding. For Gadamer "interpretation is not a timely act later and further the understanding, however, comprises always interpret, and therefore the interpretation is the explicit understanding" (Gadamer, 1998, p. 459).

In Psychology, for example, when we encourage the exercise of thinking about ways of being, in order to highlight the senses involved, it opens horizons of understanding.

The proposition of the chapter to think about the psychotherapeutic exercise encourages a hermeneutical thinking way understood from itself, every time the experience if it goes to be analyzed. Otherwise, clinical exercise resign if the legitimacy of standards to regulate our relations. The understanding of exercise resumes activity be attentive to the phenomena in their manifestation horizons contributing with other analytical propositions other than the hegemonic.

CONCLUSION

From the brief explanation suggested in this chapter, psychotherapy of inspiration in Heidegger's hermeneutic phenomenology discusses topics such as health and disease processes inherent to man's living conditions. These themes provide openness to possibilities, allowing a trial relations, free and committed way ethically. For illness and health are admitted as opportunities to reflect on our lifestyles and our relationships.

The reader should also consider that the ethical exercise enables ponder the co-belonging between being-self and others, effective freedom. Thus, in the presence of existential limits of finitude condition and illness phenomena or opening exercise the chances that health presents the human finds its own possibilities of living in the world.

REFERENCES

Foucault, Michel. (2010). *A hermenêutica do sujeito:curso dado no Collége de France* (1982-1982) (Hermeneutics of the subject: given course at the College de France (1982-1982)); tradução Márcio Alves da Fonseca, Salma annus Muchaail – 3 ed. (Translation Marcio Alves da Fonseca, Salma annus Muchaail – 3rd ed.) - São Paulo: Editora WMFMartins Fontes.

Gadamer, Hans-Georg. (1998). *Verdade e Método* (Truth and Method). *Traços Fundamentais de uma hermenêutica filosófica* (Fundamental features of a philosophical hermeneutics). Editora Vozes 2 edição (Publisher Voices 2nd edition). Petrópolis. Rio de Janeiro.

______. (2007). Hermenêutica em Retrospectiva. *Heidegger em Retrospectiva* (Hermeneutics in Retrospective. Heidegger in Retrospective). Volume I. Editora Vozes. Petrópolis. Rio de Janeiro.

______. (2011). *O caráter oculto da saúde* (The hidden nature of health). Tradução de Antônio Luz Costa – 2 ed. (Translation Antonio Light Coast – 2nd ed) - Petrópolis, Rio de Janeiro: Vozes.

Heidegger, Martin. *Seminário de Zollikon* (Seminar Zollikon). In: Medard Boss. Tradução de Gabriela Arnold e Maria de Fátima de Almeida Prado. EDUC (Translation Gabriela Arnold and Maria de Fatima Almeida Prado. EDUC). Petrópolis, Rio de Janeiro: Vozes. 2009.

______. (2012). *Ser e tempo* (Being and time). Tradução Fausto Castilho (Translation Fausto Castilho). Campinas, SP: Editora da Unicamp; Petrópolis: Editora Vozes.

BIOGRAPHICAL SKETCH

***Name*:** Danielle de Gois Santos.

***Affiliation*:** Manoel Messias dos Santos and Maria José de Gois Santos.

***Education*:** Master's degree in psychology, doctoral researcher in psychology.

***Address*:** Judge Maynard Avenue, 1005, Aracaju, Sergipe, Brazil.

***Research and Professional Experience*:** Clinical care, university professor, researcher.

***Professional Appointments*:** Researcher in psychology CNPq.

***Honors*:** Master's in psychology.

***Publications Last 3 Years*:**

Santos, Danielle de Gois. Reflexões heideggerianas na clínica: por uma ética cotidiana (Heideggerian reflections in the clinic: for an everyday ethics). *Clínica and Cultura*, v. 3, p. 1-1, 2014.

Santos, Danielle de Gois; Roberto Novaes de Sá. A existência como cuidado elaborações fenomenológicas sobre clínica psicoterapêutica (The existence as care phenomenological elaboration on psychotherapy clinic). *Revista da Abordagem Gestáltica (Impresso)*, v. 19, p. 01, 2013.

Santos, Danielle de Gois; Santos, D. A.; Lima, L. A. O.; Mendonça Filho, M. C. C. Trajetórias de Socialização: modos de dizer e de fazer aproximando agentes prisionais, internos e comunidade (Trajectories of socialization: ways of saying and doing approaching prison officers, internal and community). *Scientia Plena*, v. 5, p. 117701-1-117701-7, 2009.

In: Psychotherapy
Editor: Dominic Brewer

ISBN: 978-1-63485-226-5

Chapter 2

PSYCHOSEXUAL THERAPY IN PERSPECTIVE: STRATEGIES FOR THE NON-SPECIALIST COUNSELOR

David L. Rowland*, PhD, and Brittany Gutierrez, MA
[1]Department of Psychology, Valparaiso University,
Valparaiso IN, US

ABSTRACT

Psychosexual therapy may present special challenges for the health care provider. The sensitive nature of the problem as well as the specific issues themselves may leave some therapists uncertain regarding their ability to effectively counsel individuals having such problems. This chapter provides an essential understanding of sexual issues so therapists can confidently address problems with both knowledge and strategies that help individuals and/or couples overcome sexual difficulties. The chapter gives an overview of the sexual response cycle so the therapist acquires an understanding of the salient issues surrounding sexual problems and discusses classification of sexual problems based on the Diagnostic and Statistical Manual of Mental Disorders. Then, application of standard therapeutic procedures in the treatment of sexual problems is provided, including examples of specific sexual problems in both men and women. Benefits and limitations of psychosexual therapy for the treatment of sexual problems are discussed, with attention to those that ameliorate

* Corresponding author: david.rowland@valpo.edu.

specific sexual response problems vs those that target overall sexual relationship satisfaction. A final section considers the value of using a therapeutic strategy that combines a psychosexual approach with the use of effective pharmacological and/or biomedical options.

Keywords: psychosexual therapy, sex therapy, sex counseling, DSM-5, cognitive, emotion, mindfulness, behavioral, couples, men, women

INTRODUCTION

Ironically, it took the increased use of pharmacological solutions for men's and women's sexual problems to help clarify the role of psychosexual therapy in the treatment of these problems. If nothing else, the past two decades have taught us that while medical interventions can reduce physical symptoms, psychosexual counseling is often needed to help "heal" both the person and the relationship.

We are still far from having a complete understanding of basic human sexual response, let alone sexual dysfunction. For example, we do not completely understand why some men seem unable to control or delay their ejaculation, or why some women have difficulty reaching orgasm. But the field of sexology has reached the point where it can at least identify and describe the problems, and implement strategies that help men and women overcome various types of sexual impairment and, equally important, restore the quality of the sexual relationship.

This chapter is written for a broad audience that includes not only non-specialist therapists, clinicians, and even physicians whose patients/clients raise concerns about their sexual well-being, but also the patients/clients themselves and their partners. Although some sexual problems invariably require the attention of a specialist, many others can be handled adequately by the non-specialist assuming (1) he or she already has training as a therapist or clinician, and (2) he or she has acquired a reasonably broad understanding of men's and women's sexual dysfunctions—their etiologies, diagnoses, and treatments. Meeting these assumptions ensures that the therapist's general counseling skills are contextualized and tailored to meet the needs of clients who express a sexual concern or difficulty.

It is indeed the second assumption above that has provided the impetus for this chapter. Many therapists may not feel qualified or comfortable dealing with the sexual problems of clients. This chapter not only provides general frameworks for thinking about sexual response and sexual problems, but also demonstrates how various counseling approaches can be applied to sexual problems by the non-specialist. This chapter does not include counseling strategies for other types of sexual disorders, for example, those dealing with gender identity or gender dysphoria, or those pertaining to the paraphilias (inappropriate behaviors or objects of sexual interest).

Organization of This Chapter

In the first part of this chapter, we provide a description of sexual response as currently conceived, along with its various components. These "stages" of sexual response, although not part of the awareness of patients' experience of sexuality, provide helpful clinical delineations in terms of identifying where a particular sexual problem lies, specifying the probable etiology, and deciding on an appropriate treatment strategy. Although sexual problems are generally similar across men and women, the prevalence of problems differs substantially by sex—hence various problems are more common among men, other problems more common among women, and some worsen with age (see Table 1). As part of this discussion, we describe the problems associated with the various stages of sexual response, including diagnostic categories from the Diagnostic and Statistical Manual of Mental Disorders (DSM-5) and the International Classification of Disease (ICD), while also noting that many problems related to sexual response/performance may not necessarily exceed the threshold for classification as a dysfunction. As examples, in order to qualify for a diagnosis of premature ejaculation according to DSM-5, a man has to ejaculate within about 1 minute of penetration (American Psychiatric Association, 2013). Yet many men feel that they become aroused too easily and lack of sense of control over delaying their ejaculation, although their latency to ejaculation may extend beyond one minute. In a similar fashion, a woman may be able to reach orgasm during masturbation, but she has difficulty reaching orgasm during sexual activity with her partner (e.g., intercourse). Although she may not meet the classification for female orgasmic disorder, psychosexual therapy can address various couples' issues that might result in a more sexually satisfying relationship.

In the second and third parts of this chapter, we briefly review a number of the major counseling strategies available to the therapist, and discuss how they can be applied to men or women having sexual problems. Some strategies work better for some types of sexual problems than others; some are used more frequently with one sex than the other; and some are aimed at directly affecting sexual response, while others are more focused on finding ways to improve overall communication and sexual satisfaction. Although within our limited discussion we are unable to address each of these points in detail, we do provide broad guidelines and trends regarding optimal implementation of various counseling strategies with respect to sexual problems.

The final part of this chapter examines the evidence supporting the use of combined therapies, namely a biomedical/pharmaceutical treatment used in conjunction with psychosexual therapy. As noted above, pharmacological approaches have proven highly effective in addressing some problems related to sexual response. In those instances, the pharmacological approach may be sufficient, but in many others, adherence and psychological and relationship benefits can be maximized with the addition of brief counseling.

UNDERSTANDING THE SEXUAL RESPONSE CYCLE

The sexual response cycle is characterized by the sequence of responses and changes in the human body—physically, psychologically, and emotionally—when becoming aroused and engaging in sexual activity. This response "cycle" has been delineated primarily for the convenience of researchers and clinicians—few people would parse sexual response into various discrete stages based on their phenomenological experiences with a partner.

The first and most widely influential model of sexuality was proposed in 1966 by Masters and Johnson (Masters and Johnson, 1966), a four stage linear model of human sexual response. After studying over 10,000 participants' physiological responses, they identified four successive stages: excitement, plateau, orgasm, and resolution. In men, the *excitement* phase is characterized by increased respiration, heart rate, and blood pressure, with concomitant engorgement of penile blood vessels (vasocongestion) to generate erection, increased muscle tension (myotonia), nipple hardening, and testicle enlargement. In women, there is an engorgement and erection of the clitoris, uterus, and labia majora and minora. Uterine position elevates slightly and vaginal lubrication begins. The *plateau* phase represents an intensification of the excitement phase with blood flow, heart rate, and breathing increasing and then stabilizing, while muscle tension may increase and spread to other areas of the body. In women lubrication increases in and around the vagina as it expands and darkens. The uterus elevates fully and sensitivity increases in the clitoris. In men, Cowper's glands may secrete pre-seminal fluid from the penile opening as the testes are drawn into the scrotal sac. *Orgasm*, though not necessarily always reached, is the climax of sexual excitement. Orgasm is characterized by the subjective feeling of euphoria and relief of pressure with involuntary muscle contractions in the pelvic region and throughout the body. The muscle tension in women involves contraction of the muscles around the uterus and vagina. Orgasm in men is a two stage autonomic response. The first stage is emission where the seminal vesicles, vas deferens, and prostate cause the urethral bulb to fill with seminal fluid, with closure of the bladder neck to prevent urine leakage. In the second stage, expulsion, muscles around the penile base contract and expel semen. The final phase of the model is *resolution*, characterized by a return to baseline. Blood pressure and respiration return to a pre-arousal state as muscles relax and blood flow to genitals decreases. Masters and Johnson described a refractory period for men during which they were incapable of immediate or successive orgasm; however this period was presumed to be much shorter in women, who were capable of multiple orgasms in a short time period. Although groundbreaking at the time, Masters and Johnson's model was soon criticized for being too narrow a conceptualization regarding the complexity of sexual response and, although it had been intentionally physiologically focused, it did not account for the phenomenological and emotional aspects of sexual relationships, which are both important aspects of sexuality and motivating for partners.

Several years later, Kaplan (1977) and Leif (1977) independently suggested a tri-phasic model of sexual response: desire, excitement, and orgasm. This model represented an important step forward in the recognition of psychological factors and desire. Kaplan retained the linear model and believed desire was a prerequisite for the following sexual excitement and orgasm phases; that is, there must first be an interest to engage in sexual activity before the physiological changes of arousal occur. The very concept was created to incorporate the various aspects of sexual response beyond the physiological, including emotional, psychological, and cognitive. In the desire stage, an individual must wish/want to become aroused, having the motivation to seek and/or respond to sexual stimulation and enjoyment. In Kaplan's revised model, the excitement and orgasm phases represented a compilation of the excitement, plateau, orgasm, and resolution stages characterized by Masters and Johnson.

These traditional models of sexual response, while influential and enduring, were not without criticism. Beginning about two decades ago, four major criticisms of the traditional models of sexual response were offered. The first was the assumption that sexual desire is an automatic and spontaneous drive towards sex; the second was the idea that desire and arousal are separate entities, thereby giving rise to the third criticism, namely the presumption of a linear model sequencing through first desire, then arousal, and finally orgasm. The final criticism concerned the strong emphasis on the physiological components of the cycle, at the cost of minimizing the importance of the relational, contextual, and psychological aspects of human sexual response. Although not all the above criticisms were fully justified (e.g., Kaplan's model exhibited substantial flexibility and could well accommodate the first and last criticisms), oversimplification of Kaplan's model by subsequent researchers and clinicians made revision inevitable. As a result, recent changes have been made to the conceptualization of human sexual response, particularly vis-à-vis sexual desire in women.

One new model is grounded in the drive theory research of Clark Hull and Kenneth Spence in the 1950s and 60s (Hull, 1951), which has resurfaced in the incentive-motivation model proposed by Toates (2009). This model views desire as sometimes (though not always) the result of arousal, rather than vice versa. In this view, desire is an acknowledgement of psychological and physiological changes induced by arousal which then leads to sexual action; specifically, the motivation to respond physically precedes the incentivizing stimuli. Compared with earlier models, this approach can better account for the various differences in sexual experiences across individuals and sexes.

Another model that has garnered attention is the "circular" model of sexual response recently proposed by Basson and others (2001). The model arose from a particular emphasis on women's sexual experiences, with clinicians noting that many women appear to lack "spontaneous" sexual desire and therefore may end up being pathologized for having a lack of desire when, in fact, their condition represents a normality among women. In this non-linear model, desire occurs in response to stimuli, creates arousal and a further desire to continue this arousal. The arousing stimuli may be sexual or nonsexual, with intimacy, love, and other relational factors playing a role. The circular model avoids a dichotomy between the physiological and the psychological, with the woman initially "idling" in a neutral state (no desire, no arousal). Given the appropriate context, she may seek or respond to stimuli, activating the cycle. This response can build on itself from various stages, with desire increasing arousal or increasing stimulus-seeking and furthering the cycle. A focal point of this circular model is the recognition that physical and psychological satisfaction may create or increase emotional intimacy as well as deliberate inclusion of the contextual components sometimes involved in sexual response. These elements, though developed to explain the female experience, can be applied to either sex, and can explain the response of individuals who either have or lack spontaneous sexual desire, because the model establishes several ways desire can play into the stimulus-arousal loop. In essence, then, this model is an amalgamation of elaborated traditional models that gives greater acknowledgement to the significant role of the relational and emotional factors in partnered sexual response.

SEXUAL DYSFUNCTIONS

Despite past and recent revisions to the understanding of the sexual response cycle, sexual dysfunctions are generally tied to one or more of the phases mentioned above—desire, arousal, and orgasm. That is, broadly speaking, disorders are typically related to problems with sexual interest or desire, problems with physiological (such as erection and lubrication) and/or psychological (e.g., not feeling aroused) arousal, and problems reaching orgasm, either too quickly or only after prolonged stimulation or not at all (see Table 1 for estimated prevalence of dysfunctions in men and women). A major rationale for retaining the multiple phase approach to the understanding of sexual response lies in the fact that the etiology and treatment of problems for each of these phases may be different. At the same time, the interrelatedness of the phases of the sexual response cycle means that problems in one part of the sexual response cycle may be related to problems in another part. For example, the inability of a man or woman to achieve orgasm may be heavily influenced by insufficient arousal during sexual activity. Therefore, while the theoretical divisions of desire, arousal, and orgasm are useful in terms of treatment options, counselors should remain aware of the strong connections between such phases and avoid a reductionistic approach.

Sexual dysfunctions are classified by the Diagnostic and Statistical Manual of Mental Disorders, fifth edition (DSM-5) (American Psychiatric Association, 2013) and International Classification of Diseases, tenth edition (ICD-10) (World Health Organization, 2007) diagnostic criteria. The current sexual dysfunctions are as follows, with DSM classifications listed first, followed by the ICD classification in parentheses: 302.71 (F52.0) Male Hypoactive Sexual Desire Disorder; 302.72 (F52.21) Erectile Disorder; 302.75 (F52.4) Premature Ejaculation; 302.74 (F52.32) Delayed Ejaculation; 302.72 (F52.22) Female Sexual Interest/Arousal Disorder; 302.76 (F52.6) Genito-Pelvic Pain/Penetration Disorder; and 302.73 (F52.31) Female Orgasmic

Disorder. It should be noted that distinction may be made between someone who meets threshold diagnostic criteria for a sexual dysfunction and someone who is suffering from a sexual problem that results in frustration, dissatisfaction, and sometimes avoidance of intimacy but does not meet the criteria for dysfunctional status. Either type of individual could potentially benefit from treatment, although only a person from the former category would be diagnosed with a DSM 5 disorder.

Table 1. Sexual dysfunctions and their prevalence*

Sexual Dysfunction	Estimated Prevalence Range	Effect from Aging
Low Sexual Desire	15-25%	↑↑
Erectile Dysfunction (ED)	10-25%	↑↑↑
Premature Ejaculation (PE)	5-30%	↑
Delayed Ejaculation (DE)	5-15%	↑↑
Female Sexual Desire dysfunction (FSD)	15-40%	↑
Female Arousal dysfunction (FAD)	10-30%	↑
Genito-Pelvic Pain Disorder (GPP)	16-28%	?
Female Orgasmic Disorder (FOD)	10-25%	↓

*Aging tends to increase the prevalence for most sexual problems. In men, the ED increase is often associated with disease (e.g., cardiovascular); increases in PE and DE are sometimes related to medical or psychological issues leading to acquired problems. In women, increases are most often related to menopause. The mild decrease in FOD tends to be an early aging effect (between 20 and 35 years) that results from increased sexual experience.

Male Sexual Dysfunctions

Low sexual desire (clinically, HSDD)[1] is characterized by a lack of fantasies and/or sexual desire, whether caused by a lack of internally-driving factors (such as hormones) or by de-motivating partner/context factors. Sexual desire can be affected by life stressors, like disease, stress, crisis, and psycho-behavioral problems, situations that relegate sexual interest and activity to a lower priority. Relationship issues can also result in low sexual desire. Lack of

[1] HSDD is specifically a psychiatric diagnosis, whereas low sexual desire may have many and varied etiologies; as a result, we prefer to refer to the more general condition of low sexual desire.

sexual attraction and partner sexual dysfunction may contribute to diminished interest/desire level toward a specific partner; however, in such instances, the sexual interest/desire may be channeled or directed in other ways (masturbation, erotic materials, another partner, etc.). One cause of *general* low sexual desire in men is biological: Low levels of androgens have been implicated in low sexual desire in men, in particular both circulating "free" and bound testosterone. Also noted as having an effect on sexual desire are prolactin, due to its effects on testosterone, and neurotransmitter levels, such as elevated serotonin and histamine or low dopamine. Nevertheless, relationship and partner factors also play significant roles in men's sexual desire toward their specific partner and should not be overlooked (Rowland, 2012).

Erectile dysfunction (ED) is the difficulty in acquiring and/or maintaining an erection. Erectile response requires vascular and neural systems to be functioning properly, as erection results from neurologically-controlled vasodilation, increased blood flow to the penis, and decreased venous drainage due to increased pressure at the base of the penis. Thus, any process that disrupts vascular integrity may result in erection problems. Diabetes, hypertension, heart disease, and other symptoms of metabolic disorder (e.g., obesity) can be an underlying cause for erectile dysfunction, and, inversely, erectile dysfunction may serve as a warning sign for such medical conditions (Lewis et al., 2010). Medication, recreational drugs, and physical trauma can also disrupt erectile response, along with abnormalities within the endocrine systems, including deficient androgens, elevated cortisol, and so on. Psychological factors—particularly feelings of performance demand—can cause or intensify erectile problems. Given the aging male population in the US, the prevalence for organic-based ED is probably higher than that of psychogenic ED, but segmentation of these populations is seldom carried out in epidemiological studies so actual prevalence of each type remains unknown. Other life factors, including general stress from life events, psychological trauma, and partner and relationship issues can affect erectile function. Even when organic factors are suspected in the cause of ED, significant issues related to self-efficacy, self-confidence, and the relationship with the partner may exacerbate the problem. Furthermore, problems with erection could stem from low levels of sexual interest and desire.

Premature Ejaculation (PE) is the tendency to ejaculate rapidly, within about one minute of penetration, and is characterized by the man's inability to delay the event. Men with a lifelong history of PE typically have no clear etiology, either psychological or pathophysiological—that is, there are no obvious cardio-vascular, biochemical, or anatomical abnormalities. In cases when PE occurs as the result of a pathophysiological issue, it is often related to another medical condition, such as lower urinary tract problems, hyperthyroidism, and occasional cerebrovascular accidents. In such cases, the PE typically develops later in life after a period of normal functioning. Some drugs have also been known to occasionally induce PE, including amphetamine, heroin, and pimozide, but these effects are generally rare. Most drugs that affect the orgasmic phase delay or inhibit ejaculatory response (Rowland, Touhy and Humpfer, 2014).

Men naturally/inherently vary in their ejaculatory response latency, showing something of a positively skewed distribution. In this respect, very short ejaculatory responses may simply represent a natural variation rather than a pathological condition. Nevertheless, such short latencies often cut short the sexual and emotional intimacies enjoyed during intercourse, and thus may lead to individual and partner distress and dissatisfaction. Although no psychogenic causes can be linked directly to PE, several may exacerbate the condition. Anxiety, for example, may induce sympathetic control earlier within the sexual response cycle, triggering the ejaculatory response "prematurely" before the man is fully aroused. Furthermore, as with any sexual failure, PE is often characterized by a clear pattern of ruminating negative thoughts which can maintain or worsen the condition.

Delayed Ejaculation (DE) is a difficulty reaching ejaculation whereas inhibited ejaculation (IE) is a complete inability to reach orgasm. Similar to PE, DE/IE often has no clear pathophysiological causes, although when it does, it is usually evident from the man's medical history (Perelman and Rowland, 2008). Biomedical explanations for DE/IE have included low penile sensitivity (e.g., from aging), high ejaculatory threshold, or disease or injury affecting the sympathetic or somatic nervous systems. Damage to the lower pelvic region and spinal cord from trauma, injury, or disease along with impaired neural integrity can contribute to ejaculatory dysfunction. Psychosocial and relationship issues often play a significant role in DE/IE. For example, men who experience a discrepancy between their expectation of sex (perhaps established through fantasy or erotic materials) and their experienced reality of sex may suffer from DE. Men who masturbate frequently or use techniques (e.g., vigorous with greater pressure) that differ substantially from penetrative sex may feel under-stimulated. Factors such as partner attractiveness, sexual orientation, and the particular sexual activity (e.g., oral, vaginal, anal) may diminish the man's overall level of arousal, thereby affecting his ability to reach orgasm.

Female Sexual Dysfunctions

Female sexual interest/arousal disorder (FSIAD) is characterized by a lack of sexual interest/desire and arousal. This condition often has a complex etiology involving a combination of pathophysiological, psychological, and/or relationship factors (Brotto and Basson, 2014; Meana, 2010; Laan and Both, 2011). Although DSM now classifies sexual desire and sexual arousal as a single disorder, therapists often diagnose and/or treat them separately, particularly if the problems have clear and different etiologies—the rationale for recently combining them stems from women's lower likelihood of viewing desire as separate and distinct from arousal, and also from the fact that desire and arousal problems sometimes share common etiologies and treatment strategies. Deficiency of estrogen, which plays a crucial role in the maintenance of function and structure of vaginal tissue, is associated with decreased vaginal lubrication and blood flow, but may also, along with androgen levels, play a role in women's desire. Elevated prolactin, due to nursing or pathophysiology, may also disrupt sexual function. Parasympathetic and motor dysfunction from conditions such as spinal injury and multiple sclerosis impact arousal, as can neurovascular problems resulting from heart disease and diabetes. Psychological and relationship factors—typically more important to understanding arousal and desire problems in women, yet more individualized and difficult to specify—can include life stressors (that result in re-arrangement of priorities), relational issues, poor body image, and negative thoughts and attitudes about sex. Depression and anxiety are also largely implicated, as well as past sexual trauma (e.g., abuse) which may inhibit desire or arousal, or both.

Genito-Pelvic Pain/Penetration Disorder refers to chronic pain from sexual activity which is not caused from lack of vaginal lubrication. Not much is known about this disorder as most data regarding this dysfunction are correlational (Weijmar Schultz et al., 2005). Dyspareunia, that is, genital pain, has been correlated with low estrogen and with vaginal or vulvar infections. Tissue damage from any source—surgery, trauma, abuse, and disease—can cause genital pain; muscular spasms can increase pressure and thus intensify pain. Pregnancy, oral contraceptives, obesity, and pelvic musculature may play a role. Psychological factors appear to play a less significant role, being more likely to exacerbate the problem than to cause it. Thus, catastrophizing, hypervigilance, and negative affectivity surrounding the dysfunction may magnify the effects of the problem substantially.

Female orgasmic disorder (FOD) is an enduring delay or inability to reach orgasm under "normal" sexual circumstances, including adequate stimulation and time (Graham, 2010; Prause, 2012). Nearly half the women having problems reaching orgasm do not become sufficiently aroused, and therefore the problem lies in the arousal rather than orgasmic phase. Few obvious biological factors contribute to FOD, but relevant factors include medications, endocrine anomalies (e.g., estrogen imbalance or adrenal dysfunction), nervous system damage, serious illness, and physical injury. Often, psychological factors offer a better understanding of FOD. Relational and psychological issues, the latter including low self-confidence and conflicting thoughts, can interfere with the orgasmic function. Anxiety is also a contributing factor, and because women sometimes blame themselves for inadequacies (including those in bed), the performance demand and associated anxiety may increase, further perpetuating the problem. In many instances, the lack of orgasmic response can be traced back to contextual factors—simply inadequate time and lack of sufficient foreplay. In other instances, however, women may experience difficulty reaching orgasm even with adequate stimulation, during either partnered sex or masturbation.

TREATMENT TOOLS/APPLICATION

A trained therapist has many tools at his/her disposal, most of which have use within the context of psychosexual therapy. Thus, the basic methods and techniques used with clients in addressing their various problems are also relevant when working with individuals or couples experiencing sexual problems. An important initial step for the therapist is to normalize the situation—clients are often reluctant or embarrassed to discuss their sexual problems, so receptivity, understanding, sensitivity, and support on the part of the therapist are critical to convey. Furthermore, the therapist can convey to the client that sexual complications, although sometimes more embarrassing to discuss, have the potential to be treated in a manner similar to other disorders or challenges.

A second step is to determine the nature and scope of the problem (identifying the specific sexual problem as noted in the previous section), assessing its severity and link with other sexual response issues, and exploring etiological pathways.[2] (See Tables 2a/b for examples of medications that often affect sexual response). A related step for the therapist is to ascertain the extent to which the problem is sexual, relational, or both sexual *and* relational. Generally, the rule is that significant relationship issues need to be addressed and resolved before dealing with sexual problems.

Table 2a/2b.[3] Putative effects of common medications on sexual function in men (2a) and women (2b). For men, problems with arousal are mainly related to erectile dysfunction; problems with orgasmic function may include either delayed/inhibited or decreased intensity of orgasm. For women, problems with arousal may include lack of lubrication as well as vaginal atrophy; problems with orgasmic function may include either delayed/inhibited or decreased intensity/quality of orgasm

2a. Effects on men			
Substance Type	Desire	Arousal/erection	Orgasmic Function
Anti-hypertensives		X	
Antidepressants	X	X	X
Antipsychotics	X	X	X
Anti-epileptics			X
Cancer Treatments	X	X	
Immunosuppressive		X	
Antiandrogens	X	X	X
Steroids	X	X	
Alpha Blockers			

2b. Effects on women			
Substance Type	Desire	Arousal/lubrication	Orgasmic Function
Anti-hypertensives	X	X	X
Antidepressants	X	X	X
Antipsychotics	X	X	X
Anti-epileptics	X		X
Oral Contraceptives	X?	X?	
Cancer Treatments		X	X
Antiandrogens	X	X	X
Alpha Blockers			

2 More detail regarding the evaluation and diagnosis of sexual problems, including resources and assessment tools, can be found in the twin companion volumes by Rowland (2012) and Meana (2012).

3 Adapted from Australian Prescriber, 36(2), 42-45, 2013.

In this next section, we review a number of common therapeutic approaches that may be helpful for individuals or couples struggling with sexual issues. We note, in advance, that a number of these approaches are aimed at improving overall sexual confidence and satisfaction rather than "fixing" a dysfunctional (often, genital) response *per se*. Nevertheless, several specific behavioral approaches may not only improve overall satisfaction but sexual response as well. Although medico-pharmacological interventions may resolve certain symptoms quickly, they do not always address collinear problems (particularly psychological and relationship issues). No medication should be considered a panacea; therefore, the utilization of psychotherapeutic strategies can be both relevant and helpful.

Cognitive Therapy

Cognitive psychosexual therapy is concerned with perceptions, feelings, and interpretations related to and during sexual activity. The concept behind cognitive approaches is that anxiety, faulty beliefs, and distorted thinking are responsible for many of the sexual problems individuals and couples experience. Clients, for example, may experience any number of faulty beliefs which are often predicated and exacerbated by miscommunication and/or incorrect assumptions on the part of the client him/herself, or based on the client's perceptions of his/her partner. A man with PE, for example, may believe sexual intercourse must last a long time or involve continuous thrusting to satisfy a partner; likewise, a woman who is not adequately lubricated or receives mixed messages about her sexual role may develop low levels of arousal or genital pain. Cognitive therapy targets these faulty cognitions, any unhelpful coping mechanisms, and encourages open communication within the sexual dyad (Rowland and Cooper, 2011). Distorted thoughts can further negative beliefs or emotions and can even lead to the anticipation and expectation of problems. Once a client experiences what may have been an isolated or situational response, anxiety over what may happen the next time can lead to a belief that recurrence of the problem is inevitable, intensifying the problem and perhaps even leading to avoidance of sexual intimacy altogether (Rowland and Adamski, 2015). Thus, these distorted beliefs can cause clients to focus more on their fears and anxiety than the sexual activities in general. "Spectatoring," a common problem among those experiencing sexual difficulties, occurs when the man or woman is so preoccupied with observing and evaluating his/her own performance that he or she fails to fully engage in and enjoy the physical and psychological sensations of the sexual act. Spectatoring can lead to a loss of arousal during sex and generate self-defeating thoughts, such as "I am a failure at sex, there's no point trying or continuing because I will always have this problem" (Meston, 2006).

A number of specific cognitive approaches probably familiar to most therapists might be used to deal with distorted beliefs, including: Desibels, Counters, Self-Instruction, and Rational-Emotive Behavioral (REBT). In the *Desibels* techniques, clients challenge distorted beliefs by asking questions regarding the dysfunctional condition (what is the evidence for this, what's the worst that could happen, etc.) (Hackney and Cormier, 2009). *Counters* has the client create counter statements to the distorted beliefs. These statements must be succinct, believable, and grounded in reality; they are created by the client and subsequently rehearsed so he/she can own and accept them as truths (McMullin and Giles, 1998). *Self-Instructional* training has the client replace negative and self-defeating thoughts with positive ones (Rowland and Cooper, 2011). *REBT* is founded on the idea that a person's past experiences shape his/her beliefs and thought patterns, yet it is concerned with the client's feelings and emotions as well (Ellis, 1992). REBT thus acknowledges the negative attitudes and emotional impact caused by cognitive distortions (Rowland and Cooper, 2011), and attempts to identify and replace such faulty beliefs with more objective and accurate assessments.

As is apparent, the purpose of cognitive approaches in the treatment of most sexual dysfunctions is not to focus on elements of dysfunctional response but to improve a client's disposition toward the dysfunction and improve his/her self-efficacy and attitude (Rowland and Adamski, 2015). Cognitive approaches seek to improve the client's thoughts and internal dialogue regarding the particular sexual dysfunction and sexual activity in general. By having clients target their own self-defeating beliefs and challenge their faulty perceptions, cognitive approaches help give the client a sense of control and improve the outlook toward sexual activity.

Emotion-Focused Therapy

Emotion-focused therapy uses the negative emotions experienced by individuals suffering from sexual dysfunction as useful sources of information. Typically a short term psychosexual therapy, it considers emotion as integral to information processing (Greenberg, 2004). The three goals of emotion focused therapy are the following: to increase emotional awareness, regulate emotion, and replace negative emotions with positive ones. Just as in cognitive therapy, where clients must develop awareness of faulty or negative thought patterns surrounding their sexual dysfunction, in emotion-focused therapy, the emotional fallout of the sexual problem must also be acknowledged as a first step in treatment. Thus, whether a client or couple has been denying negative feelings about the sexual dysfunction, or has been overwhelmed with negative emotions because of it, the therapist needs to work with the client/couple to recognize this emotional component of the problem and then begin to address it: The goal is to help the client regulate his/her emotions and reduce anxiety related to the sexual problem.

Strong negative emotions can in fact make a client feel powerless and worsen the sexual problem (Meana, 2012). An emotion-focused approach assumes that while many emotions may be associated with a particular experience of sexual dysfunction, one or two usually predominate. These strong negative emotions then are likely to overpower potential positive feelings about the situation. However, these negative emotions—commonly anger, sadness, shame, or guilt—must be dealt with before the client can move past them and experience the positive emotions typically associated with sexual intimacy (Rowland and Cooper, 2011, 2016). Some helpful concepts to aid clients in emotional regulation are the acknowledgements that: emotions are within the person's control; therefore emotions can be altered toward a more positive and productive feeling; one does not have to surrender to the first emotion felt; and emotions are just that, emotions, not statements of facts (Meana, 2012). That is, emotions, as a matter of course, are subjective; they do not necessarily reflect the outer world accurately. Moreover, emotions are generally "filtered" through previous experiences, and so the therapist may need to work with the client to uncover and address unconscious premises accepted by him or her as objective truth.

As in cognitive based therapy, anxiety is acknowledged in emotion-focused therapy, but in the latter, anxiety is treated as an emotional state rather than a cognitive process. By using the four concepts described above, the client can begin to gain control over negative emotions such as anxiety. Because emotion is often processed/experienced before cognitive thoughts (Greenberg, 2004), the awareness and regulation of negative emotions may need to occur before a client can potentially acknowledge faulty or self-defeating beliefs surrounding the sexual dysfunction. In other words, clients are often required to address emotional issues before they can productively reframe faulty cognitions.

The client is further advised that, realistically, negative thoughts and emotions will continue and should be anticipated— they are an unavoidable consequence of being human under stressful conditions. Some negative thoughts will be distortions that are acknowledged as normally occurring and worked through, and some will not be distortions, either exaggerated responses or not based on the reality of the situation. Some negative emotions may be a natural result of dissatisfaction with a sexual experience that for whatever reason—biological, relational, and psychological—was beyond the client's control. As in any couples experience, the expectations of each partner will not always align with one another, nor will expectations always meet with the reality of a situation (Meana, 2012).

Behavioral Therapy

Behavioral approaches to psychosexual therapy view sexual dysfunctions as a learned, likely conditioned, behavioral response to stimuli. Since so much of the sexual response is physiological, a behavioral focus tends to explore the manner in which the sexual stimuli are presented and thus received. This response can then be changed by conditioning the client to have more "appropriate" or desired responses through stimulus control and response. Behavioral approaches to sexual psychotherapy are often focused on the direct actions of the client and partner. Techniques include alternating stimulation and withdrawal, a focus on partner arousal or needs, specific intercourse positions and maneuvers, and masturbatory exercises. Behavioral approaches also make use of different movement or relaxation of muscles, deep breathing or breathing from the diaphragm, and movements with less muscular tension (Carufel and Trudel, 2006).

Examples of popular behavioral technique used in treating premature ejaculation include Masters and Johnson's "stop-squeeze" (1970) and Kaplan's "start-stop" (1979) techniques. Kaplan's technique involves penile stimulation up to the point near orgasm (and before ejaculatory inevitability), then stopping stimulation, and beginning the process again. In this manner the client gains some desensitization while becoming more aware of his physiological responses at various points along the sexual arousal continuum (Rowland and Cooper, 2016). Similar behavioral techniques are often used in men with delayed ejaculation and in women with both arousal and orgasmic disorders. Regarding the latter, by engaging in specific behavioral techniques to stimulate the clitoris, such as with vibrators, woman positioned on top, etc., women can become more aware of their physical sexual response, pleasure, and arousal. Consistent with this approach, it is often useful to have women (in particular) become more familiar with their genitals. As female genitalia are not as readily perceived as male genitalia, and as societal messages about female genitals and self-exploration often leave women unsure of their bodies and insecure in exploration (Meana, 2012), by having women engage in masturbation and self-exploration, often with a mirror, they can become more comfortable with their bodies so as to learn how they respond to different types of stimulation to various parts of their genitals. For both men and women, after exploring on their own, they can then move to focusing on responses during stimulation in a partnered experience. Behavioral techniques for arousal-based dysfunctions in partnered experiences then often involve building on foreplay and either speeding up or slowing down the client and partner (Rowland and Cooper, 2011). Behavioral techniques are useful in treating sexual dysfunction not only because they address the physical responses of sexual activity, but also because they create distance from any personal faults in the client, as the focus is on the behavior to be modified rather than the individual him- or herself.

Mindfulness Therapy

Mindfulness is a form of self-awareness, an internal, passive awareness of the present and ongoing experience. Mindfulness therapy teaches the client to focus on his/her thoughts, reactions, and emotions in a non-judgmental and accepting manner. Mindfulness builds on many of the same ideas as the behavioral and cognitive approaches, with the core tenet of experiencing without passing judgement often being very apropos in therapy for sexual dysfunction (Brotto and Basson, 2014). Mindfulness sexual therapy is particularly concerned with the bodily sensations and awareness of the five senses, in the present moment (Mize and Iantaffi, 2013). Furthermore, the mindfulness view of sexual therapy negates the idea that sexual intimacy is merely a means to an end, particularly by men who tend to be goal-oriented and often engage in sex with the goal of orgasm. Women, on the other hand, often engage in sexual intimacy from a partner-orientated perspective, with intimacy itself as an endpoint (Basson, 2001). Thus, mindfulness stresses the idea that the sexual act and intimacy may themselves be endpoints, rather than avenues through which one may achieve orgasm.

Mindfulness therapy also teaches clients to be aware of their bodily sensations and response. Understanding the importance of this process years ago, Masters and Johnson (1970) developed sensate focus techniques still used with regularity in psychosexual therapy today. Sensate focus enables participants to learn to experience sensual touch in a non-demanding context. Typically, sensate focus begins with participants engaging in non-genital touch, with the goal to increase communication and trust, while not focusing on erection and/or orgasm as expected endpoints. After some time, clients are directed to begin genital touch, while still avoiding orgasm as the goal (Masters and Johnson, 1970). The practice of mindfulness and sensate touch is useful in counteracting the "spectatoring" that is often characteristic of sexual performance anxiety. Individuals learn to experience sexual touch without expectation or demand. For non-medically-based sexual dysfunctions, including ED and PE in men, and FSIAD and FOD in women, mindfulness techniques and sensate focus can be quite effective, but even when a sexual problem such as erectile dysfunction is organic in nature, mindfulness can help clients become more aware of their bodily sensations and responses.

As noted above, mindfulness has proven quite useful in the treatment of a number of male sexual problems. The anxiety and shame associated with these problems can create a self-perpetuating cycle, so the non-demanding nature of sensate focus techniques is particularly helpful because it teaches men that sensual contact and the associated pleasure may be endpoints in and of themselves, rather than specific genital responses. Absent a particular genital response as an end goal, the fear of failure is eliminated—as there is no goal at which to fail. Mindfulness teaches a sense of personal responsibility for one's sexual desire, pleasure, and performance.

Mindfulness is also helpful in the treatment of Female Sexual Interest/Arousal Disorder, having been found to increase sexual arousal, desire, satisfaction, and lubrication. Sexual distress and orgasmic difficulties tend to decrease while overall sexual responsivity increases (Brotto and Basson, 2014). Mindfulness allows women to explore their emotional and bodily responses to sensual touch by focusing on themselves rather than a partner or particular aim. The approach grounds the client in what is currently happening, exploring what is pleasurable, what is not, and where their boundaries reside.

Couples Therapy

Couples therapy often involves the collection of all the previous tools. The main objective of couples' therapy is not the use any one particular technique, but rather in having the sexual partners join together in the exploration and treatment of sexual dysfunction (McCabe et al., 2010). The main tenet of a couples-focused treatment toward sexual dysfunction is that regardless of whoever is experiencing impaired functioning, the couple as a whole is affected, as the sexual relationship is impaired. Whether the dysfunction is situational or global, and whether the individual has only experienced impairment with the current partner or all previous partners, the current relationship plays an important part in working through the sexual problem. By working with the couple together, each partner is able to express relevant feelings and responses. Each is able to aid the other in understanding what works, what does not, and what to do to create realistic expectations.

Couple-focused therapy has at its core open communication and shared responsibility. This approach takes away the sting of shame, the fear of disappointed expectations, and the confusion of miscommunication and assumptions. Couples therapy has been used effectively for both male and female dysfunctions: desire/arousal, pain, erectile, and orgasmic/ejaculatory disorders. The strength in couples therapy lies in the partnership, leaving the couple open to choose whatever particular treatment tools fit best, with the benefit of having a partner and support system built into treatment. Couples therapy can focus on communication, role playing, and specific behaviors as they relate to the particular sexual dysfunction, say premature ejaculation; or it might focus on broader relational issues, including intimacy, interactions, and overall satisfaction. Whether through functional or dysfunctional interaction, communication always plays a key role. Many of the faulty cognitions, insufficient coping mechanisms, and negative attitudes and emotions experienced by individuals suffering from sexual dysfunction are related to misperceptions—about the self, the partner, and the interactional/relational components of sexual activity.

While all the previously mentioned psychosexual therapies can involve the partner, at least to some extent, in some instances the participation of the partner is important. For example, a cognitive approach in couple's therapy would have the couples analyze the overt and covert messages partners are expressing. A behavioral approach would have couples examine their behaviors and resulting individual and partner responses, while an alternative approach would have the couple unite as a team to account for the dysfunction

(Rowland and Cooper, 2016). While all of these strategies might be implemented on their own, the goal of a coupled approach is to strengthen the overall relationship, help the pair understand the respective roles each plays, and help them work together to overcome the dysfunction. Couples therapy is also useful in allowing the therapist and couple to address issues outside the sexual dysfunction that might impede progress, for example, erection problems that result from the negative interactional style of the couple, or low desire that may reflect the emotional distance of a lagging relationship rather than a specific sexual issue.

THE CLIENT-THERAPIST RELATIONSHIP

As therapists know, counseling content, techniques, and methodology constitute an important element of the therapeutic process. Equally important to treatment outcomes, however, is the nature of the client-therapist relationship—the therapist must actively partner with the client (or couple) in order to maximize treatment efficacy. This partnership may be accomplished through a number of techniques as outlined below (Choca and Van Denberg, 1996).

The first and often most effective technique is giving unconditional positive regard, showing empathy for the client and his/her problem, and being sincere throughout the therapy process. This support—important to the treatment of any problem—is especially critical in psychosexual therapy, given the sensitive nature of the issue and often accompanying embarrassment. Being honest and empathic with the client demonstrates the commitment and understanding of the therapist and increases the chances of compliance and participation. Empathy can be expressed through reflective listening and open, non-judgmental communication (Rowland and Cooper, 2011). The understanding expressed by the therapist to the client can also increase the client's satisfaction.

The next technique is Motivational Interviewing (MI). As the above conditions are met, it is necessary to understand the importance of clear and thoughtful communication. Motivational interviewing is a patient-centered style of prompting behavioral changes by encouraging an intrinsic desire to work through inconsistencies and by helping clients set goals for change (Rowland and Cooper, 2016). MI improves the client's openness to the process of change by examining various patterns—behavioral, cognitive, relational, and emotional—and thus typically increases the client's commitment to therapy. As part of MI, various communication techniques between client and therapist can be developed so as to strengthen the client's dedication to treatment and exploration of interaction patterns, including working through resistance, building self-efficacy, and recognizing inherent discrepancies.

"Recognizing discrepancy" refers to the process of working through where the client currently is and where he/she would like to be in the future (Bundy, 2004). Recognizing this discrepancy allows the client to understand the need for change, by first setting then achieving the goal (Rowland and Cooper, 2011). While behavioral response changes related to the sexual dysfunction (e.g., increased ejaculatory latency or orgasm frequency) are often primary goals, other goals may include ones related to affective and relationship issues, for example, improving communication with the partner, regulating negative emotional states, and addressing and changing faulty cognitions.

Client resistance is not uncommon during therapy, and so a strong partnership with the client becomes critical during such periods. This resistance may develop for any numbers of reasons, including unrealistic client/partner expectations, impatience, relationship issues, or when the sexual dysfunction has become part of an unhealthy coping mechanism; it may also be intensified by medical issues (Rowland and Cooper, 2011). Whatever the reason, when resistance occurs, the therapist must understand the causes, avoid pushing too hard for change, and eventually, in conjunction with the client, develop a tailored approach to the client's particular resistance style (Rowland and Cooper, 2011). Through such partnering, the therapist not only empowers the client but also increases his/her commitment to change (Bundy, 2004).

Finally, building clients' self-efficacy is important because it enables them to deal with many of the aforementioned problems, helping them feel they can handle the challenge before them and successfully commit to and make changes. Increasing self-efficacy allows them to understand that while the counseling may be guiding and encouraging them, the client him or herself is ultimately responsible for the change (Bundy, 2004).

BENEFITS AND SHORT-COMINGS OF PSYCHOSEXUAL THERAPY

Psychosexual therapy approaches have both benefits and shortcomings. See Tables 3a/b for outcome possibilities for specific therapies used in the treatment of various sexual dysfunctions. On the positive side, and in comparison with biomedical approaches, psychosexual approaches often focus on improving the overall sexual relationship and communication, a key component to achieving sexual satisfaction. In some instances, benefit may include improved sexual responsiveness as well, as with some orgasm and arousal phase issues.[4] Furthermore, through therapy, the client and/or couple has access to a newly-developed set of cognitive, emotional, and relationship coping skills that may be useful in future situations when relapses occur. Therapy can allow for and encourage the client/couple to begin enjoying sex again and focusing on the sensations and experience, rather than focusing on the mechanics or perceived short-comings (McCabe, 2001). Finally, these strategies for improvement avoid chemical use—important to some patients—as well as the adverse effects that typically accompany it.

Perhaps the most relevant disadvantage is that for some types of dysfunctions, the therapies themselves do not improve sexual performance; thus, those dysfunctions that involve a significant biological component generally do not respond well to psychosexual approaches. Furthermore, psychosexual therapies—although generally deemed effective in achieving broad outcome goals—do not have the benefit of having been rigorously tested (not only due to a lack of large sample studies, but also to the fact that psychosexual therapy approaches do not lend themselves well to randomized, placebo controlled analysis). Therefore, their efficacy is more difficult to quantify, sometimes making them less attractive to potential clients, particularly given the required commitment of time and, often, personal resources.

COMBINATION APPROACHES

One of the more promising treatment options for sexual dysfunctions lies in the use of combination therapy. Combination therapy brings to bear biomedical treatment options in conjunction with psychological ones, an approach that has been found to be effective especially with those sexual dysfunctions having a significant biological component. A biomedical approach involves medication, physical therapy techniques, or even surgical

[4] For more details about the specific therapeutic processes for each of the male and female dysfunctions, including various assessment instruments, the reader is referred to *Sexual Dysfunction in Men* (Rowland, 2012) and *Sexual Dysfunction in Women* (Meana, 2012).

intervention. Medical treatment often relieves potential underlying conditions causing the dysfunction or helps create more advantageous physiological conditions for unimpaired sexual response, while the psychosocial treatments address a client's responses, any developed potential coping mechanisms, effects from having lived with a sexual dysfunction, and improved interaction with the partner. Perelman (2003) has mentioned the idea of "coaching," or targeting certain behaviors or possible impediments to pharmacological treatments clients may receive (Brotto, 2015). Evidence for the overall effectiveness of combination therapies comes from a number of studies, most recently a meta-analysis which found combination therapy superior to either type alone, regardless of the particular psychological treatment approach (couple, CBT, individual, etc.) (Schmidt, Munder, Gerger, Fruhauf, and Barth, 2014). Combination therapy can involve the merging of different styles of psychosexual treatment as well. As in couple's therapy, where the merging of different techniques is considered important, combination therapy can involve a medical approach of pharmacological intervention for physiological issues while behavioral techniques offer more effective stimulation, and emotion and cognitive techniques target maladaptive feelings and thought processes.

An example of the important role that counseling can play is seen in the recent FDA approval of the drug Flibanserin for the treatment of low sexual desire in women. Clinical trials revealed that the drug had a latency period of about 8 weeks, suggesting it would take some time for the drug to exert its positive effects (Brotto, 2015). In such cases, it could be beneficial for users to receive some form of counseling to address potential concerns and relationship issues, thereby increasing treatment efficacy and the likelihood of continued medication usage. Yet, even when the pharmacological treatment is fairly fast acting (e.g., medical treatments for ED or PE), complementing biomedical treatment with psychosexual therapy may offer significant benefits. Impairment of sexual functioning typically causes significant distress personally and interpersonally, affecting the individual's self-efficacy and disrupting his/her role/relationship with the partner. Psychologically-based treatments can offer a balance, allowing the client a chance to manage other aspects surrounding the sexual dysfunction but also to learn how to integrate treatment and level of functioning into their lives and relationship, leading to more sexually satisfying experiences. Thus, as with most disorders, a holistic approach may provide the optimal way to conceptualize and treat sexual problems. In such cases, supplemental counseling need not be extensive and lengthy, but rather focused specifically on identifying and addressing issues that might serve as impediments to the effectiveness of the biomedical treatment, whether cognitive, emotional, behavioral, or relational, with the goal of reframing and replacing negative/ counterproductive strategies with positive/productive ones.

Table 3a. Male Sexual Dysfunction Treatment Type Effects

Dysfunction	Cognitive	Emotion-focused	Behavioral	Mindfulness	Couples
Low Sexual Desire					
Cognitive-emotional reframe	X	X		X	X
Sexual satisfaction	X	X	X	X	X
Sexual performance			X		X
Better relationship					X
Erectile Dysfunction (psychogenic)					
Cognitive-emotional reframe	X	X		X	X
Sexual satisfaction		X	X	X	X
Sexual performance			X	X	X
Better relationship					X
Premature Ejaculation					
Cognitive-emotional reframe	X	X		X	X
Sexual satisfaction	X	X	X	X	X
Sexual performance			X		X
Better relationship					X
Inhibited Ejaculation					
Cognitive-emotional reframe	X	X		X	X
Sexual satisfaction	X	X	X	X	X
Sexual performance			X		X
Better relationship					X

Finally, even when relationship and cognitive/emotional factors are not issues, ongoing adherence to medication has been identified as a significant problem in the biomedical treatment of sexual dysfunction. Specifically, attrition rates for medical treatments for ED and PE sometimes exceed 50%, often because patients are dissatisfied with the outcomes, specifically vis-à-vis the cost/benefit ratio (Brotto, 2015). In such instances, brief counseling can assist the client or couple with setting realistic treatment goals, identifying alternative and supplemental ways to enhance the treatment efficacy, providing a greater repertoire of behaviors that might enhance mutual sexual satisfaction, and establishing reasons for adhering (or not adhering) to medication use. Of course, combination therapy is not possible when no prescribed pharmacological treatment is available for the specific sexual problem, but when such options are possible, therapists and clients might consider such an approach in order to maximize benefits (Levine, 2015).

Table 3b. Female Sexual Dysfunction Treatment Type Effects

Dysfunction	Cognitive	Emotion-focused	Behavioral	Mindfulness	Couples
Female Sexual Interest/ Arousal Disorder					
Cognitive-emotional reframe	X	X		X	X
Sexual satisfaction	X	X	X	X	X
Sexual performance			X		X
Better relationship					X
Genito-Pelvic Pain					
Cognitive-emotional reframe	X	X		X	X
Sexual satisfaction	X	X	X	X	X
Sexual performance	X		X		X
Better relationship					X
Female Orgasmic Disorder					
Cognitive-emotional reframe	X	X		X	X
Sexual satisfaction	X	X	X	X	X
Sexual performance			X		X
Better relationship					X

CONCLUSION

On those occasions that clients or couples raise issues about sexuality within the context of counseling, the therapist need not necessarily provide a referral to a specialist. Most therapists possess the therapeutic tools and skills that can be used for the successful treatment of sexual problems or dysfunctions. Understanding the basic elements of sexual response, how response and problems differ across the sexes, and the possible etiologies of the problems enables the therapist, from an informed perspective, to offer guidance, help, and support to the client. Typical cognitive, behavioral, emotion-based, mindfulness, and couples therapeutic approaches can be applied by therapists as they assist clients in managing and/or recovering from a sexual problem. Such therapies also offer the potential to improve psychological functioning through increased self-confidence and self-efficacy; and they can improve relationship functioning through improved communication and support from the partner. In those instances where a strong biological cause is implicated—and for which a biomedical treatment exists—therapists and clients should discuss the option of a combination approach that draws on both biological and psychological remediation/treatment.

REFERENCES

Basson, R. (2001). Human sex response cycles. *Journal of Sex and Marital Therapy, 27*(1), 33-43.

Brotto, L. A. and Basson, R. (2014). Group mindfulness-based therapy significantly improves sexual desire in women. *Behaviour Research and Therapy, 57*, 43-54.

Brotto, L. A. (2015). Flibanserin. *Archives of Sexual Behavior, 44*(8), 2103-2105.

Bundy, C. (2004). Changing behaviour: Using motivational Interviewing techniques. *Journal of the Royal Society of Medicine, 97*(44), 43-47.

Carufel, F. D. and Trudel, G. (2006). Effects of a new functional-sexological treatment for premature ejaculation. *Journal of Sex and Marital Therapy, 32*(2), 97-114.

Choca, J. P. and Van Denburg, E. J. (1996). *Manual for Clinical Psychology Trainees*. 3rd edition. Levittown, PA: Brunner/Mazel.

Diagnostic and statistical manual of mental disorders: DSM-5. (2013). Washington, D.C.: American Psychiatric Association.

Ellis, A. (1992). Group rational-emotive and cognitive-behavioral therapy. *International Journal of Psychotherapy, 42*, 63-80.

Graham, C. A. (2010). The DSM diagnostic criteria for female orgasmic disorder. *Archives of Sexual Behavior, 39*: 256–270.

Greenberg, L. (2004). Emotion Focused therapy. *Clinical Psychology and Psychotherapy, 11*, 3-16.

Hackney, H. and Cormier, L. S. (2009). *The professional counselor: A process guide to helping*. Boston, Mass: Allyn and Bacon.

Hull, C. L. (1951). *Essentials of behavior*. New Haven: Yale University Press.

ICD-10 international statistical classification of diseases and related health problems. (2005). Geneva: World Health Organization.

Kaplan, H. S. (1979). *Disorders of sexual desire and other new concepts and techniques in sex therapy*. New York: Simon and Schuster.

Laan, E. and Both, S. (2011). Sexual desire and arousal disorders in women. *Advances in Psychosomatic Medicine, 31*, 16–34.

Leif, H. (1977). Inhibited sexual desire. *Medical Aspects of Human Sexuality, 7*: 94-95.

Levine, S. B. (2015). Flibanserin. *Archives of Sexual Behavior, 44*(8), 2107-2109.

Lewis, R. W., Fugl-Meyer, K. S., Corona, G., Hayes, R. D., Laumann, E. O., Moreira, E. D., Jr., Rellini, A. H. and Segraves, T. (2010). Definitions/epidemiology/risk factors for sexual dysfunction. *The Journal of Sexual Medicine, 7,* 1598–1607.

Masters, W. H. and Johnson, V. E. (1966). *Human sexual response*. Boston: Little, Brown.

Masters, W. H. and Johnson, V. E. (1970). *Human sexual inadequacy*. Boston: Little, Brown.

McCabe, M., Althof, S. E., Assalian, P., Chevret-Measson, M., Leiblum, S., Simonelli, C. and Wylie, K. (2010). Psychological and interpersonal dimensions of sexual function and dysfunction. *The Journal of Sexual Medicine*, *7*,327-36.

McCabe, M. (2001). Evaluation of a cognitive behavioral therapy program for people with sexual dysfunction. *Journal of Sex and Marital Therapy*, 27, 259-271.

McMullin, R. E. and Giles, T. R. (1998). *Cognitive-behavioural therapy: A restructuring approach.* New York: Grune and Stratton.

Meana, M. (2010). Elucidating women's (hetero) sexual desire: definitional challenges and content expansion. *Journal of Sex Research, 47(2-3)*: 104-122.

Meana, M. (2012). *Sexual dysfunction in women*: *Advances in psychotherapy-evidence based practice*, Cambridge, MA: Hogrefe.

Mize, S. J. and Iantaffi, A. (2013). The place of mindfulness in a sensorimotor psychotherapy intervention to improve women's sexual health. *Sexual and Relationship Therapy, 28*(1-2), 63-76.

Perelman, M. A. (2003). Sex coaching for physicians: Combination treatment for patient and partner. *International Journal of Impotence Research, 15*, Suppl 5, S67-S74.

Perelman, M. and Rowland, D. L. (2008). Retarded or inhibited ejaculation (male orgasmic disorder). In Rowland and Incrocci (eds). *Handbook of Sexual and Gender Identity Disorders*, Wiley Press, pp.100-121.

Prause, N. (2012). The human female orgasm: critical evaluations of proposed psychological sequelae. *Sexual and Relationship Therapy, 26*: 315-328.

Rowland, D. L. (2012). *Sexual dysfunction in men: Advances in psychotherapy-evidence based practice.* Cambridge, MA, USA: Hogrefe Publishing.

Rowland, D. and Adamski, B. (2015). Sexual dysfunction, epidemiology of. *International Encyclopedia of the Social and Behavioral Sciences, 21*, 711-721.

Rowland, D. and Cooper, S. (2011). Practical tips for sexual counseling and psychotherapy in premature ejaculation. *The Journal of Sexual Medicine, 8*, 342-352.

Rowland, D. and Cooper, S. (2016). Treating men's orgasmic difficulties. In Zoe Petersen (ed) *Handbook of Sex Therapy*. Wiley-Blackwell, in press.

Rowland, D. L., Touhy, A. and Humpfer, J.(2014). An integrative approach to the treatment of premature ejaculation. *Current Reports in Sexual Health, (6)*2 124-135.

Schmidt, H. M., Munder, T., Gerger, H., Frühauf, S. and Barth, J. (2014). Combination of psychological intervention and phosphodiesterase-5 inhibitors for erectile dysfunction: A narrative review and meta-analysis. *The Journal of Sexual Medicine, 11*(6), 1376-1391.

Toates, F. (2009). An integrative theoretical framework for understanding sexual motivation, arousal, and behavior. *Journal of Sex Research, 46*(2-3), 168-193.

Weijmar Schultz, W., Basson, R., Binik, Y., Eschenbach, D., Wesselmann, U. and Van Lankveld, J. (2005). Women's sexual pain and its management. *The Journal of Sexual Medicine* 2: 301–316.

BIOGRAPHICAL SKETCH

Name: David L. Rowland (first author)
Affiliation: Valparaiso University, Department of Psychology
Education: Ph.D.

Address: 1001 Campus Drive, Valparaiso IN 46383 USA

Research and Professional Experience: 40 years as researcher and author regarding the study of clinical populations with sexual problems. Professional appointments include: Professor of Psychology, Editorial Boards of 3 journals, prior editor of the Annual Review of Sex Research, co-founder and co-editor, *Journal of the Mind and Medical Sciences.*

Publications:

Over 150 publications, including refereed articles, books, and book chapters.

Dr. Rowland's research has focused on the understanding of sexual response and its problems in both men and women. Much of his research has taken a psychophysiological approach, attempting to understand the relationship between physical/physiological sexual response and the psychological experience of the response and dysfunction within clinical populations.

In: Psychotherapy
Editor: Dominic Brewer
ISBN: 978-1-63485-226-5

Chapter 3

MEETING THE EMOTIONAL NEEDS OF PEOPLE WITH INTELLECTUAL DISABILITY AND TRAUMA

Patricia Frankish*
Pat Frankish Psychology and Psychotherapy Consultancy,
Kirton Lindsey, Gainsborough, UK

ABSTRACT

This chapter will explore the emotional needs of people with intellectual disabilities, looking at methods for identifying the issues and ways of working to enable progress to be made. A treatment and support model is provided that has been shown to be effective in clinical settings. The approach is novel and yet to be researched with more participants.

Keywords: trauma, emotional development, intellectual disability, psychotherapy, attachment

* Corresponding author: Patricia Frankish, Dr. Psychology and Psychotherapy Consultancy, Artemis House, 25, High Street, Kirton Lindsey, Gainsborough, DN21 4LX, UK. E-mail: Pat.frankish@patfrankish.co.uk.

Introduction

Traditionally people with intellectual disabilities were seen to have a deficit in their emotional world as well as their cognitive world. Over the last 20 to 30 years there has been a growing body of evidence that this is not the case. The emotional development is subject to the same tensions and issues as for those without disability, with the same potential consequences. What does seem to be the case, however, is that the lack of ability to cognitively process experiences can lead to delayed emotional development and/or extreme responses to traumatic events (Sinason 1992).

It follows from the above situation that there is a need to address the emotional developmental needs of individuals with disabilities, as well as to address the consequences when things go wrong. People who have been described as exhibiting challenging behaviour are re-framed as people with complex needs as a result of trauma and in need of trauma-informed care (Frankish 2016). This chapter will go on to describe some key features of trauma-informed care (TIC) and a theoretical understanding of why it is needed. There will also be reference to ways of assessing the difficulties and designing interventions to match. From the beginning it is noted that attachment needs are the significant factor (Gerhardt 2004), and individual psychotherapy may be a requirement for effective complex treatment plans.

Emotional Development

We all grow up in relation to other people. We all have attachment needs (Bowlby 1979). People with disabilities are no different but may be put in situations that hinder the establishment of secure attachments. The baby who has to stay in hospital without mother, of who has to have alternative care from the beginning, will have difficulty forming a strong attachment to one person. We know that the development of self occurs through the process of relating to one person, then two, then three, and lastly to a group of people (Fairbairn 1952). This can be interrupted for any of us and will have consequences in later life on mental health and personality development. For the child with a disability the pathway can be more treacherous, leading to expressions of behaviour that can put more pressure on families and lead to them choosing alternative provision for their child. Joan Bicknell (1983) referred to the handicapped family when a child with disability is identified.

The life-style changes significantly, with lots of professional visitors, tests, questions, search for a cure and such like. The divorce rate is much higher in couples who have a child with disability. If the stage of acceptance is reached there can be good progress towards accepting the disabled child as a valued member of the family, different but still loved and wanted. If it isn't reached the family becomes dysfunctional with the emotional consequences that would be expected.

Mahler (1975) established a measurable model of emotional development, building very much on the work of Winnicott (1973) and this model has been adapted for use with people with disabilities. In turn their work used the attachment model first proposed by Bowlby (1979). The presence of a significant other is shown to be essential for the development of the sense of self as a good-enough person and this is just as relevant for the disabled child as it is for any child. Winnicott wrote about the need to be able to rationalise in order to reach the more mature emotional developmental stage of separation. This requires cognitive ability and it often the stumbling block to the full establishment of the self as an independent being. Mahler refers to the rapprochement crisis occurring at the time of individuation, that point at which being separate can be tolerated with manageable anxiety.

Many people who exhibit challenging behaviour after early childhood end up in institutional care. They become too difficult for parents to manage at home, and too disruptive of the lives of their siblings. As the primary cause of their difficult behaviour is often an attachment issue, sending them away is potentially going to make matters worse. But it can be understood as families become trapped in a situation they cannot resolve. If we can help them to understand what is happening and provide an intervention to help to resolve the primary issue, it may be possible to help everyone in the family. If alternative living is the best option, then it is vital that support staff are trained to understand the problems and provide support in a manner that is likely to be helpful.

Traumatic Events

Sometimes there are traumatic life events on top of the primary difficulty of the disability and the normal trials of growing up. Trauma is very idiosyncratic. In other words, what is traumatic for one individual, may not be traumatic to another. We have to look at how someone responds to an event to ascertain the impact. Many events of childhood are not noticed by anyone, and it can be many years before the specific event is recognised as having been traumatic for the individual. If the person with a disability is not able to speak or explain what has happened it makes it even harder to work out what it was. And, of course, sometimes the trauma will be abuse, physical, sexual or emotional, and the perpetrators will have an investment in making sure it is not known or understood. Sadly the occurrence of abuse of people with disabilities is high, which will be for a variety of reasons, some of which will be because they are not seen as reliable witnesses to what has happened to them, some by families who cannot bear the pain of having a disabled member and all the other reasons for why perpetrators do what they do. On top of this is the trauma associated with abandonment and rejection, which can be felt if it happens emotionally even if not physically. Being unloved is painful and children who grow up feeling unloved will be harmed and suffer trauma.

WORKING OUT WHAT HAS HAPPENED

Faced with someone who is hurting themselves, trashing their room, or attacking others, the question is inevitably, "why?" If the behaviour has persisted for many years it is harder to find an initial trigger. Behavioural interventions would begin by analysing the behaviour and looking for a trigger to start it, or a consequence that is seen as a gain. So, for instance, an individual who is desperate for physical contact may explode in order to be restrained. It is unlikely that they want to be restrained but it is the only way they have found that works to achieve the aim of being held. For most people it is unlikely that they have this as a thought, more a pattern of desperation followed by relief when someone else takes control and there is the comfort of feeling held.

Finding the answer to the question "why?" can take some time. The first stage is to establish the level of intellectual disability so as to ascertain the assessments that might be helpful. People with mild to moderate disability can usually do some drawing and answering questions types of assessment, whereas non-speaking people will more likely need an observational methodology. Looking at the history can be helpful but often the behaviour has persisted for so long that the initial cause is lost in the mists of time. What follows is an approach to answering the question and then some ideas of how interventions may be planned to address the needs shown up by the assessment.

Assessment of Emotional Needs

For people with mild disabilities it is useful to secure responses to the Brief Symptom Inventory (Derogatis 1975, 2004) which has norms for people with disabilities. This gives an indication of the severity of the distress in terms of models of mental illness. The score can indicate "caseness" which is an indication for a therapeutic intervention. This is a self-report measure so is subject to the usual problems of "faking-bad" or "faking-good." It is because of the uncertainty with self-report that the next stage is to look at projective tests. With these tests there is no right or wrong answer so they give a deeper and more accurate understanding of the individual. They do not, however, give scores that can be compared so they do not lend themselves to being useful in research. The results apply only to the individual.

House, Tree, Person

The House, Tree, Person test is recommended for use with anyone who can hold a pencil and make marks on paper. Some of the drawings may not be recognisable as a house, tree and person, but the way they are drawn and the differences between each one can be analysed. It is essential that it is not introduced as the house, tree person test or the testee will draw all three on one sheet of paper. The sheets are offered separately with a request to draw each one in turn. The house is indicative of basic security and groundedness, the tree of ego development and the person, identity. The pictures are analysed for similarity in size and style as well as content. If all three pictures are central to the page, drawn with confidence and recognisable as what they are with all features present, then there are no issues. This is rarely the case for someone referred for assessment. We see pictures of houses with no door, lots of windows, phallic chimneys, tiny or huge, drawn with shady lines or harsh black lines. There are tiny trees, ones with cut off tops or no roots, some with additional holes or creatures. Then people which are stick figures, no body, one arm or leg bigger than the other, some tiny, some filling the page.

Some examples of interpretation would be that a house with no door indicates feeling trapped inside or refused entry, a tree with no roots indicates denial of the past, and stunted top suggest stunted ego development, probably caused by trauma. A tiny person, especially if house and tree are ordinary, indicates low self-esteem or feeling invisible. There is a short handbook available from www.frankishtraining.co.uk which gives more information. Learning to use the test can be facilitated by FT.

Some drawings can be barely recognisable and an example would be scribble. But if the scribble is different for each picture, it indicates an understanding of the task by the individual and their attempt to show you what they are feeling. The quality and style of the scribble can give an idea of how they feel about their basic safety, ego development and sense of self.

Object Relations Technique

The next projective test to consider is the Object Relations Technique (ORT) (Philipson 1988). This test uses ambiguous pictures to elicit stories which are then analysed. The instructions are to say what is seen, what they think is happening and what they think will happen next. It is used more with a non-disabled population but has been found to be useful with this client group. The stories are often brief and the ability to say "what next" is limited. This latter point is useful as it shows an inability to predict consequence, which can be very useful to know when someone is displaying difficult behaviour. It is certainly useful if it has been suggested that behaviour is governed by a consequence.

The pictures are in 3 sets of 4 and 4 sets of 3. There are three each of a one person, two person, three person and group picture, then four each of a very blurred picture, four more clear and four with colour. There is then a blank card for them to tell their own story if they can. The thirteen stories are then analysed for content, looking at who is the main character in them (assumed to represent the individual doing the test), what actions are involved, if all the figures are seen (or too many) and the outcome. The information will give clear indications of gender identification, core themes of the personality, but, more especially, a pointer towards the emotional developmental stage. If there is disturbance in the pictures of a particular group it suggests that there has been a traumatic experience at that stage of their lives.

Disturbance at the one person level is consistent with failure of primary attachment. The person is isolated emotionally, not connected to other people, not able to relate and benefit from nurture and care. They are not really suitable for individual therapy but do need to be offered a non-challenging environment that they can manage that has no emotional demands made on them.

Disturbance at the two-person level shows that the primary relationship, usually with mother, was traumatic and prevented any further emotional development. They may have a diagnosis of borderline personality disorder as well as intellectual disability. They are difficult to support because they swing from good to bad very quickly, and have to spoil anything good before someone else does. This group responds well to long-term attachment based therapy.

The three-person level is associated with the stage of emotional development where the father, or second significant other, gets involved. The emotional task of this stage is to begin to be able to choose and discriminate. Competition and envy are common factors and struggles to share are evident. They are often well able to engage in lots of activities and enjoy stimulation and winning, but may have a behavioural breakdown if things are not going their way. Individuals traumatised at this stage usually do well in therapy and become able to use their abilities more productively.

Group level trauma is associated with traumatic events that have happened at a later stage, after the basic personality is largely formed, so nursery or school-age issues. The child who has been left at school or nursery all day before they are quite ready to cope with this, will show signs in their stories of distressing situations or abandonment. They respond well to having an opportunity to explore this, mainly because the trauma will be after the development of verbal skills and is likely to have a memory trace laid down. Traumatic events from the earlier stages may only have body memories or vague feelings with no clear substance, making them difficult to process, and therapy essential.

The information from the ORT gives very quick and easy access to this information in a non-traumatic way. The information gained can then inform the therapeutic intervention. Occasionally someone will reject the test because the pictures stimulate a real memory that cannot be tolerated. If that happens the test is stopped and the individual given an opportunity to explore their reaction.

Observation Method

Quite a few people with intellectual disabilities and challenging behaviour are non-verbal, and not able to do any of the assessments so far described. Margaret Mahler (1975) did some research with young children and identified from observation the emotional development stages traversed between biological birth and psychological birth. Once it was realised that the behaviours she described were also seen in severely disabled adults, it was hypothesised that these adults were, in fact, stuck in their emotional development. This led to two big questions, why were they stuck? And could they be helped to make progress?

A method for carrying out an observation and deducing the stage was developed (Frankish 1992, 2013) which arrived at a forty-minute assessment, where the observer watches for twenty seconds, writes for forty seconds, and repeats this until forty data points are secured. It takes a bit of practice but it has been found that support staff can learn to do this, although it is usually done by psychologists or teachers. Once the forty points are written they are analysed and the emotional stage identified. Mahler used six stages but the first one, symbiotic, is very rarely seen and the last, individuation, would not be present if the individual is in difficulty.

Hence four stages are used, the first being differentiation, which occurs naturally between a few weeks of life and about 8 months. Behaviours are self-referenced, including things like exploring body parts, and the immediate environment with little if any attempt to initiate contact but reacting when it is offered. The next is practicing and corresponds with the description of stereotypic behaviour. It occurs naturally between about 8 to 15 months and is associated with rapid neurological development. As each new skill becomes available it is practiced over and over again until a new behaviour becomes available. There is more activity if the significant other is present but contact is not sought, only responded to.

Practicing is followed by early and then late rapprochement. This takes about eighteen months to two years altogether and represents the move from being isolated to being connected, the serious work of establishing a self in relation to others. In early rapprochement there is the beginnings of challenges and asserting self-will. This often starts with the ability to say "no" or to run away. As confidence grows and the significant other facilitates growing independence at the right rate, the child moves into negotiation and, eventually, into being able to be separate with manageable anxiety.

From the forty data points it is possible to identify the stage at which the person observed is stuck. They will have more points in one category than the others and this is seen as the stage. Everyone has some behaviours in the other stages but one will be dominant. It is important to recognise that many non-disabled people will be stuck at the late rapprochement stage but will be able to function if they have their cognitive skills to help them to deal with their emotional reactions. People with intellectual disabilities, and traumatic impairment of their emotional self, have an emotional disability as well. In non-disabled people this would probably be labelled as personality disorder. Seeing it as emotional disability, and amenable to intervention, is more useful to the disabled person.

SUMMARY OF TESTS

Summarising the tests enables us to see that we are arriving at similar information via different routes, and these routes are the ones that the person with the difficulty will find easiest to do. Individuals who are already traumatised and distressed need to have as non-intrusive assessment as possible, so some thought needs to go into deciding which is most likely to yield results. Once the degree of cognitive impairment and emotional developmental stage are known, it is possible to design an intervention.

INTERVENTIONS

There are four elements to a successful intervention and all need to be in place. The first is a "secure base" which is somewhere to live that is safe and assured. A tenancy or placement that depends on behaviour is not secure. There needs to be an understanding and acceptance that damage will be repaired and that any incident can be recovered from and they will not be evicted. Constant moves feature in the history of people with complex needs and there has to be a decision that this will not happen.

The second is enough staff to keep everyone safe. It may be that a single-person service with three staff on duty at all times is the starting point. This is expensive but not as expensive as secure care and has the prospect of moving quickly to reductions in staffing levels.

The third element is training and support for staff. This is training in the emotional developmental model and in how to respond to incidents, including how to use restraint, should it be needed, in a therapeutic way that is not punitive. To date we have found that the initial training can be covered in a five-day course or with some of it provided on-line for people to follow at their own speed. Staff usually react very well to the ideas and are quick to want to implement them, feeling enabled by knowledge to do what is right. They are then supported by staff support meetings, offered weekly for people to attend when they can. This is a place where they can talk about the impact of working with very distressed people, explore their reactions in a safe place and make joint plans for how to address the difficulties, facilitating a coherent response from everyone.

The fourth is psychology or psychotherapy support for the client and the staff. This may include individual therapy for the client if the assessment shows this to be necessary (it usually is), and the same person can lead the staff support meetings. It is not essential for it to be the same person but it often works out to be more efficient for the psychologist or psychotherapist to attend to see the client and then meet with the staff. If the individual being supported suffers from paranoia it will be necessary for the staff meeting to happen elsewhere, at least initially.

When all of these elements are in place there is quite rapid progress. People who have been displaying the same behaviour for years, sometimes with lots of restraint and staff injuries, respond well to feeling safe and cared for and begin to be able to manage for longer between incidents and recover faster.

An Example

This example is made up of information from several people so as to ensure the confidentiality of the individuals. We will consider a young man, age 35 years, who has been in secure care since leaving a special residential school at the age of 19. He was in the school because he couldn't be managed at home. Home was a foster home, as he was taken from his natural mother age 1 year because of neglect. He went to the special residential school age 12, when he became too big and strong to be managed by his foster parents. At school he spent a lot of time in seclusion or being restrained. Several staff had been injured by him, including a broken arm, several bites and many bruises. His medication was above safe limits as prescribed by the British National Formulary and everyone was despairing that he could ever be helped. He had a number of self-injuries from banging his head and kicking doors.

We'll call him Paul for the purposes of anonymity. He was far too distressed to be able to complete the BSI, HTP or ORT so it needed an observation of him to establish where he was emotionally. His skill level had to be used to assess his cognitive functioning. He said a few words but these were simple demands for drinks or freedom. He could, when settled, engage in some play activities, and watch others. He had some favourite toys that he held on to but which could be lost in restraint or taken away if he was in seclusion. He appeared to plan to hurt people.

The observation was completed by someone he didn't know. He watched the observer all the time but made no attempt to attach, or curiosity about what she was doing. The results showed that he was functioning at the practicing level of emotional development with some earlier differentiation behaviours and a few early rapprochement behaviours. This required that an intervention should be designed to provide what is needed to support someone who is physically thirty five, intellectually probably about four years and emotionally only one year. This discrepancy between the different developmental levels is, in my experience, always found in the very distressed complex people.

It was not possible for Paul to tell us what caused his distress but the observation result pointed to his early life being traumatic and a failure of his primary emotional development. This led to him spending his life feeling the fear of a one year old who doesn't understand the world and having to survive. His fear that everyone would leave him led to behaviour that meant people had to hold him, which made him feel safer. His self-injury in seclusion came from his fear that no-one was there for him. Seeing him as a frightened one year old in an adult body helped staff to relate to him better.

The intervention needed to include all four elements. A property was identified that was large enough for him to live in (element one) with, initially, three staff because of the need to restrain (element two). It was single storey to avoid problems with stairs and a safe sensory room was included so that he could have time alone in a safe environment, and it could be used instead of restraint if he became distressed. This room was soft-lined in bright colours and had music piped to it. A care plan for the use of the safe room included the need for staff to stay in contact at all times if he was in there, so as to avoid him feeling abandoned. It was expected, and proved to be the case, that he would not have to seek the physical contact of restraint if he felt safer most of the time.

Children at this emotional age need lots of activity and a narrative of what is happening around them. Staff were taught and encouraged to think of repetitive games and activities, always explaining what was happening. They took Paul outside and showed him things growing in the garden, helping him to engage with the world around him. They had the basic training in the model and an understanding of emotional development and emotional trauma. They were then supported to respond appropriately to incidents and to remember that fear was the main emotion behind distressed behaviour (element three).

A therapist was identified to work with Paul to try to help him to make sense and be able to tolerate what had happened to him throughout his difficult life. He had never had a secure attachment figure so the first stage was to establish contact and try to facilitate an attachment. The therapist called twice a week at the same time and on the same day. Initially staff stayed present to make sure there were no attacks. They were soon able to stay outside of the room but within earshot for if they were needed. They weren't needed, as Paul very soon recognised that the therapist was there for him, was listening, and cared about what he was feeling. Some of the pre-therapy ideas of Prouty (1994) were employed, accepting that cognitively Paul was not able to engage in traditional talking therapy at that time.

OUTCOME

Within three months Paul was able to be with the therapist without staff. He was never restrained in this service, and quickly learned to use the safe room if he felt he might lose control. Sometimes he was directed to the room by staff but this gradually decreased and he was able to decide for himself. Keeping in contact with him through the door helped him to not feel abandoned and he became able to regulate his emotions and calm down.

Medications were gradually reduced to safe limits and some stopped altogether. He remained highly aroused and needed some medication to help with this anxiety. He became able to accept blood tests to check the safe levels. He once injured himself to the degree of needing to go to hospital. Five staff went with him for safety for all but he managed to stay reasonably calm and trust that people were trying to help him.

Staffing levels were reduced from two to one in eighteen months and one to one with on-call back-up within thirty months. This corresponded with his emotional growth. As he moved into rapprochement behaviours, he became able to negotiate, ask for things he wanted, respond to questions and trust that people would come back if they left at the end of a shift. Incidents of disturbed behaviour became associated with wanting something that it wasn't possible to have just then and typical of two year old behaviours.

Paul continued to have therapy and formed a good attachment with his therapist. As he grew he became able to verbalise more and to draw. His drawings indicated the early trauma. He was able to listen and accept what his therapist explained to him and to develop a sense of self that he could live with. He was always going to need to have staff and, possibly, to live alone, but there is hope that he will be able to share as he moves through the stages, closer to individuation.

Conclusion

I have tried to give a picture of a way of working that provides very distressed people with a way foreword that has hope for change. Most of the people who present as traumatised and complex have seen no progress in their quality of life for years because of a failure to identify the need. The discrepancy between cognitive and emotional development, plus the presence of trauma, is perhaps too much for professionals to face. It is hard to accept that some of the most vulnerable people in our society have suffered such neglect of their needs, and often suffered years of restraint and seclusion. This model provides a way foreword for them.

References

Bicknell, J. (1983). The psychopathology of handicap. *British Journal of Medical Psychology*, 56, 167-178.

Bowlby J. (1979 reprinted 2005) *A Secure Base – The Making and Breaking of Affectional Bonds*. Routledge Classics.

Derogartis L R (1975, 2004) Brief Symptom Inventory.

Fairbairn W.R.D. (1952) *An Object Relations Theory of the Personality*. New York, Basic Books.

Frankish, P (1992) A psychodynamic approach to emotional difficulties within a social framework. *Journal of intellectual Disability research* 36, 559-563.

Frankish, P. (2013) Measuring the emotional development of adults with ID. *Advances in Mental health and Intellectual Disabilities*, Vol. 7, Iss. 5, pp 272-276.

Frankish, P. (2013) Facing Emotional Pain – a Model for working with people with intellectual disabilities and trauma. *ATTACHMENT: new Directions in Psychotherapy and Relational Psychoanalysis*, 7, 276-282 C.

Frankish P (2016) *Disability Psychotherapy-an Innovative Approach to Trauma Informed care*. Karnac. London.

Gerhardt S (2004) *Why love matters*. Routledge.

Mahler, M., Pine, F. and Bergman, A. (1975). *The psychological birth of the human infant.* New York: Basic Books.

Phillipson, H. (1988) The use of ORT as a facilitation of motivational process: some implication for a range of applications with special reference to subliminal activation of preconscious processing. *British Journal of Projective Psychology*, 33 (1), 84-105.

Prouty, G. (1994). Theoretical *Evolutions in Person-Centered/Experiential Therapy: Applications to Schizophrenic and Retarded Psychoses.* Westport: Praeger.

Sinason, V. (1992). *Mental handicap and the human condition*; New Approaches from Tavistock. London: Free Association Books.

Winnicott DW (1973) *The Child, the Family and the Outside world.* Middlesex.

www.frankishtraning.co.uk.

Biographical Sketch

Dr Pat Frankish grew up in the grounds of a long-stay hospital where her parents worked, so was exposed to contact with vulnerable people with intellectual disabilities from a young age. She was also aware of sometimes people needing to be restrained or put into a side room, causing them to scream and be very upset. This probably sowed the seeds for her later career.

Pat married young and had three children before training as a Clinical psychologist. Before going to University she worked for a few years in the hospital where she had grown up and gained more insight into the levels of distress experienced by the people who lived there. During her first degree course she carried out a piece of research around communication aids for disabled people. Her experience in her Clinical training at Masters Level broadened her skills to include psychotherapy, and an opportunity to use these skills with people with intellectual disabilities. This led to her using the approach and developing it further in her employment. She completed training in Clinical Psychology and then a Doctorate in Psychology, together with training to teach and, more recently, in theology.

Employment has included work in all settings, from community teams, to in-patient assessment and low, medium and high security. She conducted research to explore the reliability and validity of the observational methodology and was awarded her doctorate in 2003. Since then she has gone on to provide services for people with intellectual disabilities and trauma, putting the ideas into practice, and has continued to train others and publish the work.

Pat was also active in the British Psychological Society, serving as Division of Clinical Psychology Chair and later as President of the Society. She oversaw the Occupational Standards project, the establishment of mandatory Continuing Professional Development and the Register of Psychologist Practicing as Psychotherapists. She has, more recently, become a member of the United Kingdom Council for Psychotherapy. She was a Founder Member and Chair for many years of the Institute of Psychotherapy and Disability.

In moving toward retirement, she has written more and her first single author book has recently been published by Karnac books (London).

Publications Last 3 Years:

Frankish, P. (2013) Measuring the emotional development of adults with ID. *Advances in Mental health and Intellectual Disabilities*, Vol. 7, Iss 5, pp 272-276.

Frankish, P. (2013) Facing Emotional Pain – a Model for working with people with intellectual disabilities and trauma. *ATTACHMENT: new Directions in Psychotherapy and Relational Psychoanalysis*, 7, 276-282 C.

Frankish, P. (2013) Thirty years of disability psychotherapy, a paradigm shift? *Advances in Mental Health and Intellectual Disabilities*, Vol. 7 No. 5.

Frankish P (2016) Disability *Psychotherapy - an Innovative Approach to Trauma Informed care*. Karnac. London.

In: Psychotherapy
Editor: Dominic Brewer
ISBN: 978-1-63485-226-5

Chapter 4

EXPLORING TEMPORALITY IN PSYCHOANALYSIS: REPEATING THE PAST AND FINDING THE FUTURE

Zelda G. Knight*[*], *Prof, PhD
University of Johannesburg, Johannesburg, South Africa

ABSTRACT

Traditionally little was written about the future in psychoanalysis. This chapter explores the experience of the future because without a sense of the future, patients cannot move foreword psychologically. The original Freudian idea of the compulsion to repeat has implications for how the future is experienced and conceptualised. In this chapter, the future is linked to the concept of 'potential space' and the 'what can be' experience as well as the notion of the 'return of the repressed', indicating that the future, as potential for what can be, was blocked and repressed in the past resulting in a lost future. Little emphasis has been placed in psychoanalysis on how the future is an integral part of therapy and the how the re-working of temporality leads to healing. In exploring the future, which is also linked to hope, the corrective emotional experience is seen as a way in which the future can be found and grasped and how, in therapy, the future can be conceptualised as creating a new

[*] Corresponding author: Zelda G. Knight, Prof, PhD. Department of Psychology, Faculty of Humanities, Auckland Park Campus, University of Johannesburg, Johannesburg, South Africa. E-mail: zknight@uj.ac.za.

self. I present a short case from my clinical practice to exemplify these suggestions.

Keywords: the future, potential space, the corrective emotional experience, the return of the repressed, transference

INTRODUCTION

The idea of repeating the past in the present has always captured the attention of analysts since Freud first noticed that there was an unconscious human tendency to repeat the past in the present. He termed this pattern of repetition the 'repetition compulsion' and in 1920 he described it as:

> This 'perpetual recurrence of the same thing' causes us no astonishment when it relates to active behaviour on the part of the person concerned and when we can discern in him the essential *character*-trait which always remains the same and which is compelled to find expression in a repetition compulsion of the same experiences. (1920, p. 21)

For Freud, this 'perpetual recurrence of the same thing' or the repeating the past in the present, was first clinically noted in his case of Dora. He subsequently defined this pattern of repeating the past in the present as the process of transference (1905). He also suggested that during transference the patient is unaware of this repetition and thus acts unconsciously. The patient, he also noted, re-creates actual relationships experienced in the past with him as analyst in the present. Freud (1905, p. 116) defined transferences as:

> They are new editions of facsimiles of the impulses and fantasies which are aroused and made conscious during the progress of the analysis; but they have this peculiarity, which is characteristic for their species, that they replace some earlier person by the person of the physician. To put it another way: a whole series of psychological experiences are revived, not as belonging to the past, but as applying to the person of the physician at the present moment.

Since its inception more than 100 years ago, the concept of transference has become one of the most well-known concepts within psychoanalysis but not much has been explored regarding the implication of repeating the past in the present in terms of how time for patients, specially future, is phenomenologically experienced in analysis. Stuck in a cycle of repeating the past means that the future is not always clear or possible. It is important to explore the experience of future in psychoanalysis because without a sense of the future, patients cannot move foreword psychologically.

Freud's idea of the repetition compulsion and by implication, the unconscious processes of transference, is not unique however. Several decades before, Nietzsche (1882/1974, p. 273) also described a similar idea or repeating the past and he termed it 'the eternal return of the same.' Below is a description of this idea:

> What if some day or night a demon were to steal after you into your loneliest loneliness and say to you: 'This life as you now live it and have lived it, you will have to live once more and innumerable times more; and there will be nothing new in it, but every pain and every joy and every thought and sigh and everything unutterably small or great in your life will have to return to you, all in the same succession and sequence — even this spider and this moonlight between the trees, and even this moment and I myself. The eternal hourglass of existence is turned upside down again and again, and you with it, speck of dust!'

Despite this similarity of the idea of repeating the past, it is Freud's genius who is rightly credited with working therapeutically with the phenomenon, rather than leaving it as an abstract idea, as Nietzsche appeared to have done. Freud therefore applied this concept to deepen his understanding of his troubled patients, and he recognised the value of encouraging the development of repetition, and thus transference, in service of his patients.

He did not however, refer to how the future is experienced within this repetition phenomenon and how it could be 'lost' nor did he work therapeutically with the future.

Traditionally, while reference has been made to time in the general sense in psychoanalysis (Loewald, 1972), little was written about the future in psychoanalysis. Time within Western societies was commonly viewed as linear - the 'past-present-future' and thus as something sequential and progressively onwards. However, it is now understood that the psyche does not experience time in this linear manner but shifts back and forth between these three modalities of temporality (Loewald, 1972). The future, as an aspect of experience of time, was not a common focus of the process of analysis, nor was it theoretically linked to the concept of potential space and the emergence of a new self.

What This Chapter Is About

This chapter explores temporality in psychoanalysis with an emphasis on the future as intrinsic to healing. The original Freudian idea that we repeat the past in the present has implications for how the future is experienced and conceptualised. So much of therapy is about a re-working of the past in the present, but so little emphasis has been placed on how the future is an integral part of this re-working and healing. In exploring temporality, the future has been linked to hope but in this chapter it is also linked to the concept of potential space and thus as unrealised potential and 'what can be.' In addition, it is suggested that the 'future in the past was blocked,' and thus potential in the past was 'arrested' and repressed and so the future was lost. In terms of healing, the future is viewed as an essential part of the therapeutic process in that patients must imagine a different future, perhaps even find a lost, repressed future. The idea of the experience of a different future is linked to the corrective emotional experience which presents a 'contrasting to what is expected' experience, and thus the experience of temporality is emotionally re-configured. I offer a brief case from my clinical practice to demonstrate these ideas.

Repeating the Past and Finding the Future

The original idea, proposed by Freud (1914) of repeating the past in the present was that it was a way to master what had been a loss of mastery – meaning that the repetition compulsion was viewed as a psychological act to reclaim control over the uncontrollable. Later, this aspect of repeating the past also included the idea that unconscious repressed material seeks an outlet - manifested in the familiar analytic concept of the 'return of the repressed' (Freud, 1915a and b) – and repetition was an expression of this. Freud coined the term 'the return of the repressed' to indicate the return of unconscious instinctual desires that had been denied access to the conscious mind. Such desires had to be repressed because they were thought socially unacceptably by the ego. Freud claimed that these drives would push towards release into conscious reality and return in disguised form, as the symptom, which he interpreted as a compromise between the conflicting needs of the untamed id and the reality-based ego (Freud 1896).

In addition, Freud encouraged this repetition of the past or transference, and thus the return of the repressed, and allowed himself to be formed in, and shaped by, the needs of his patients – 'to be the replacement' – which foreshadowed the object relations theories notion of, espoused by, the Winnicottian concept of 'object usage' in which the patient 'uses' the object of the analyst in order to work through the transference.

The phenomenon of repeating the past in the present has implications for how the past, the present and the future is phenomenologically experienced. In the transference, the past is unconsciously re-enacted which means that the experience of the present has layers of unconscious dynamics and it is only through the process of working through the transference that the unconscious is made conscious. The working through of the transference is the core business of psychoanalysis and it implies the past is reworked in the present so that the future is also re-configured.

Through the re-working of the past, temporality is itself re-configured, and with it, a sense of time as a blending and merging of the past with the future in the present so that time itself is not linear but circular and ever shifting. Moreover, the future in this re-orientation of the past and the present, is something that beckons a re-working too.

The idea of 'shifting experiences of time' presents the possibility of exploring the future in psychoanalysis and not just in the context of a repeating past.

The exploration of the future in psychoanalysis was associated with the notion of the patient's hope in therapy (Cooper, 2000, 2004; Mitchell, 1993; Searles, 1979). Hope became a central theme within contemporary, post-modern relational psychoanalysis (Cooper, 2004; Summers 2005, 2010) and was connected to the idea of becoming a new person, of the 'creation of a new self' and with it, new ways of being and relating to self and other (Summers, 2005, 2010). So much of psychoanalysis today is about therapeutic action and a related emphaisis on authenticity and the creating of new experiences, and to this end, the discourse of analytic change is increasingly becoming one where the analytic relationship is one of authenticity between the two participants (Aron, 1992, 1997; Benjamin, 2005; Bollas, 1989; Summers, 2005, 2012). The distinction between recovery and creation, writes Summers (2012) has broken down as the recovery of self states that have been repressed or never conscious appear as emerging states. The uncovering of unconscious material is no longer regarded as uncovering established psychic form or fully formed psychic entities but as the creation of new forms as dissociated states emerge into consciousness. Feelings and motives discovered in analysis, he continues, are not fully formed psychic entities awaiting the light of consciousness, but unformed psychic states or potential ways of being and relating (Summers, 2012, 2005). The creation of new forms of dissociated states links in with what Freud noted regarding unconscious fantasies. In the 1908 paper, "Hysterical Phantasies and Their Relation to Bisexuality," Freud dealt with unconscious fantasies in greater detail. "Unconscious phantasies have either been unconscious all along and have been formed in the unconscious; or—as is more often the case—they were once conscious phantasies, day-dreams, and have since been purposely forgotten and have become unconscious through 'repression' " (p. 161). To repress is to "purposely forget," not to simply forget, thus it is also recognised that the unconscious content was itself conscious once. This has implications for memory and the future, and the idea of new possibilities for the uncovering of the unconscious is the uncovering of new unformulated material (formed in the unconscious) and unconscious material (formed in the conscious) but now repressed.

Both forms of unconscious material can lead to the emergence of new ways of relating and being in that the 'return of the repressed is possible.' In this light, hope is for a better future or, in terms of psychic development, it is the actualising of potential, of what can be - the uncovering of a lost self (purposely forgotten) or the development of a new sense of self (formed in the unconscious), and as such, hope is what rises out of the battle between 'what was' and 'what can be.' In Cooper (2004, p. 527) states, "hope itself, in psychoanalysis, is born of the constant tug between our emphasis on understanding the shackles of the past and the notion that new experience can emerge."

In this context, the reworking of the past in the present (in the transference) is the hope for a *new experience* and the realization that, as a result, a *different* future is possible, less dominated by the haunting ghosts of the past that bind the present. What happened in the past, the painful experiences that shape and limit the present, is what also shapes and limits the future, and so, the re-working of the past, presents a different, perhaps lost, future which is not chained to this painful past. In this way, a patient's conscious dread of the future is not really about what will be, but is instead about whatever enslavement has already happened. The future becomes a possibility of what can be, free, to some extent, of enslavement. Cooper puts it well when he writes that "the patient is often like the sole surviving Japanese soldier holding down an island in the South Pacific, fighting a war that is long over without knowing it. Often a patient's awareness that the war is over is a reconfiguration of the past, reflective of the therapeutic action of psychoanalysis" (2004, p. 528). A reconfiguration of the past is the only way that a different future can be grasped.

While the repeating past is always with us, in the re-working of the past in the transference, it is re-shaped and the power of the (painful) past is lessened. A different future means a future detached from 'what was' overwhelming and enslaving.

The experience of the future in psychoanalysis can be linked to, and expressed in, the well-known analytic notion of 'potential space' (Winnicott, 1951). Potential space in the therapeutic process is defined as something 'yet to be formed,' the potential for the creation of something new in the formlessness of that space. Thus the 'yet to be formed space' can be organized around the 'yet to be' or 'what can be' which describes the future, as anything 'not yet' is the future. Using potential space is therefore working with the future in the present, or uncovering dissociated selves. Winnicott's idea of therapy as this potential space or formlessness allows for the patient's experience to become formulated, to take shape and form in the formlessness. Using potential space also re-formulates the present to be one of emerging and 'becoming' and of a future re-formed. To this end, the modern analytical space has become defined by projections into the future that require a reconfiguration of the patient's sense of temporality. Normally patients cannot conceive of new possibilities while in the throes of experiencing their problems (being trapped in the repetition of the past) and thus they do not have a belief in a future that can be different (Summers, 2005, 2012). "In a very real way, then, there is no sense of future because the horizon of the patient's life is an endless present" (p. 26).

If this notion is extended, it means that if the patient has no sense of a future, then the patient has no hope of escaping from the fetters of the past, and no hope of something new in the present. The present therefore becomes an endless repetition of the past - 'there will be nothing new in it, even this spider and the moonlight between the trees.' In this way, the inability to conceptualize a future is the inability to conceptualize something new.

The work of psychoanalysis therefore should include supporting patients to conceive of a different future, of new possibilities and thus of moving from the relentless cycles of repeating the past, where, as Nietzsche pessimistically observed, 'this life as you now live it and have lived it, you will have to live once more and innumerable times more' to *new experiences*. If we accept that the work of contemporary psychoanalysis is about new experiences (Cooper, 2004) and thus about creating new possibilities and capabilities, and this is operationalized as creating new ways of being and relating that are not based on past relational templates, the patient must therefore envision a different future. Such re-framing of temporality means that the past itself is not only re-framed but the present gains a different meaning. In other words, "The present moment gains its meaning in the trajectory towards the future, and the past gains new meaning in the context of the experience of future and present" (Summers, 2005, p. 27).

In terms of the future, I suggest that the dynamics of the past are such that 'the future in the past' was 'blocked' and the reconfiguration of the past in therapy must also mean that the 'blocked future' is unblocked and opened up.

I link this 'blocked future in the past' to the psychoanalytic theory of psychopathology, which is understood to arise from the dynamics between what the infantile psyche needs to develop and the lack of a facilitating environment (Klein, 1955; Kernberg, 1975; Freud, 1893/1966; Sullivan, 1953; Winnicott, 1965). This convergence of thwarted needs and an environment not ideally conducive to psychic development is known in Self Psychology as 'arrested self-development' (Kohut, 1977, 1984). Expressions of arrested development have been described in detail in the analytical literature, resulting in, for example, personality disorders such as the borderline or the narcissistic personality (Kernberg, 1975; Kohut, 1977). Other expressions of arrested development have also been described in the psychoanalytic literature and range from psychosis to less severe neurotic symptoms such as depression, anxiety disorders and phobias (Klein, 1955; Mitchell, 2000; Summers, 2007). In each case, these clusters of pathology are psychological symptoms which indicate that 'something is wrong.' In this state of arrested development, the infantile self experienced a block to or barrier in the trajectory of its development, or, if put in a temporal frame, a 'barrier to the future.' This barrier to the future means the 'future in the past was blocked' and potential cut off from being actualised.

If the future is linked to potential, the past becomes one of 'arrested potential.' I would suggest that this sense of 'something is wrong' is linked to an experiential sense of a blocked/lost future and thus lost potential. However, as Freud warns, nothing in the psyche is ever lost: it is repressed. The implication of repressed potential is that the future cannot be actualised. As indicated, Freud's concept of 'the return of the repressed,' expressed as psychological symptom, highlights the psyche's capacity to heal itself and this means recover lost and occluded potential. Winnicott (1951) thought that the presence of symptoms, such as depression, was a positive sign because it meant that the psyche was trying to express what had been occluded, lost or cut off. In this context, I suggest that the return of the repressed is embodied in a sense of loss of what could have been. In this regard, it becomes important for patients to recover (a lost future) and envision a new future for themselves because it is only in reclaiming the lost future, with its lost potential, that the present can be an opportunity to actualise potential.

THE CORRECTIVE EMOTIONAL EXPERIENCE AS RE-FRAMING THE PAST AND FINDING A FUTURE

As indicated, the re-framing of the present means a re-framing of the past and by implication, the present and the future as well. I suggest this re-framing of the present, past and future can be done therapeutically through the use of hope in analysis and linking hope to the 'corrective emotional experience.' Hope is for many patients, the hope for something new, a longing to change to their dysfunctional self-other relationships, and thus a hope that in this relationship with the therapist, it could be different. Hope and the future are linked just as the concept of the corrective emotional experience is linked to change. The concept of the corrective emotional experience, as described by Alexander and French (1946) is a psychological technique and agent of change and it promises a different experience (a different present) to what is expected (a repetition of the past).

In their seminal book, *Psychoanalytic Therapy: Principles and Applications*, (1946) Alexander and French challenged the prevailing assumption that the only way to bring about change in therapy was for the analyst to uncover painful childhood repressed memories (in other words revive the past) through the use of free association and interpretation. While exploring and understanding the painful past is the business of psychoanalysis, it is not the full story of what needs to be done in therapy. Contemporary psychoanalysis is not just the intellectual understanding of the past and thus an explanation of what happened, but is an *emotional experience* in the present that contributes and supports in reworking of the past.

The corrective emotional experience, as the main agent of change, was defined as the offering of an emotional experience that was contrary to, or corrective of, what patients had come to expect (Alexander and French, 1946).

In other words, a new experience. The notion of 'contrary to what is expected' is crucial in terms of how the present is experienced and the past re-worked, and by implication, the future as re-framed. Thus, in the context of the experience of a corrective emotional experience, temporality is reconfigured because such offering of what is 'not the same' (contradicting the expectation of the present) means that patients experience something new in the present, and by inference, a different (perhaps even recovered, lost) future. The corrective emotional experience opens up in the present the hope and possibility of finding a (lost) future, and of creating a different future, and thus of 'creating a new sense of self,' as indicated earlier by Summers (2005).

Husserl (1904) and later Heidegger (1926) argued that time is experienced as projected or 'thrown towards' the future, and as we move towards the future, we encounter the past which meets us in the present. Expanding and psychologizing this idea results in the standpoint that the stories of patients (the repeating of the past) can become stories of a projected future when they have an 'experience of change' in the present (through the experience of the corrective emotional experience). Once this happens, patients need to experience a different future, and instead of the focus being on the patient's narrative of 'what was' (the past) the focus may be on the narrative of 'what can be.' If the task of the analyst in this situation is to have a future vision of what the *patient can be* even if initially the patient cannot see this future (Summers, 2005), the future experience is intrinsic to the creation of a new sense of self – of 'what can be' - because without the vision of a different future there is no possibility for change.

It is recognised however, that the corrective emotional experience is controversial as it speaks to the idea that the therapist 'does something to' the patient (offer a contrary experience to what they expect) but this is not the case. While it is not the scope of this chapter to defend this concept, suffice to say that the therapeutic process is a relational process, and as such, the analyst is always 'doing something' such as offering an interpretation or becoming the object that is needed (object usage) and thus is always responding to the needs of the patient. Offering a corrective emotional experience is responding to the patient in such a way that the patient can begin to realise, or become conscious of, their own unconscious compulsion to repeat.

The Case of Marilyn: A Short Case Vignette to Illustrate the Concept of Future[1]

A short case vignette is presented to illustrate the concept of future because this relates to the potential for healing in analysis and therefore, 'moving foreword,' as opposed to being stuck in unconsciously repeating the past.

Marilyn was a young woman in her mid-thirties, intelligent, single and working in an environment that expected her to use her skills as a writer and a teacher. She had been in therapy with me for one year and her presenting problem was that she could not decide whether to leave her work and move with her boyfriend to another city and start a new life there. Moving meant that she would leave her family and friends, something she wished she did not have to do but leaving also offered the potential for a new life and new opportunities. Our psychoanalytic process had been progressing well and she was always on time, worked hard at the issues that were raised, and discussed, when relevant, details of her own childhood experiences.

She has been brought up a Catholic, and while not practising, was prone to guilt and feeling bad. Her parents were both well-educated with university degrees and working full-time. The family unit was closely-knit and caring, but Marilyn tended to be the 'parentified child' to the mother who seemed to be neurotic and highly strung with dependency traits. As therapy continued, I realised that my patient was unable to make the decision to move out or stay because it meant that either way, she would disappoint someone (the boyfriend or the family, especially the mother) and be left feeling guilty.

In one session she recalled a childhood memory of how one day the ballet was scheduled to come to town, and two tickets were bought, for her and her mother. She was excited and could not wait. On the day of the ballet however, her mother became ill and could not go. Marilyn begged the mother to find an adult friend to take her, and the mother reluctantly made a call to such an adult friend. Just as Marilyn was about to be fetched by this friend, her mother said to her, *"I'm going to be alone if you go."* The impact of that remark was profound and left Marilyn literally frozen and unable to move out the door. As a little girl, she felt intense guilt for wanting to leave, and pressure to stay, and in that moment she made a decision not to leave her mother alone, and thus she forfeited the chance to go to the ballet.

---

[1] In order to protect the identity of the client, names have been changed and certain aspects of the history and case have been altered but the essence of the encounter remains the same.

As we discussed this memory and the experience of feeling guilty for wanting to go but of remaining frozen at the doorway, and thus of meeting her mother's needs while placing her own needs second, Marilyn became conscious of how the emotional themes of this same experience in the past was now being played out. She recognised that her current dilemma regarding leaving home, and in a sense, of being frozen at the threshold of her own 'moving out.' At one point in the session, she said to me, "I hope you don't mind if I leave you when therapy is over." In that moment in the transference, history was repeating itself with me as the replaced mother. Such a question holds the anxious hope that things will not be a repetition this time in this relationship with me, and it can be different. Such a question is the deeper, underlying longing for something new. As typical of with transference-testing, she was hoping that I would not stop her leaving, and not be the controlling mother and say - 'I'm going to be alone if you go.'

We discussed her question and what my opinion meant to her, and how it seemed with me she was re-enacting her past, but at the same time, hoping that I would be okay with her leaving. Other memories emerged as we spoke and had similar themes of her needs being put second, of feeling guilty and of others as needy.

The temporal experience of transference is that the present for Marilyn was an endless repetition of the past. But the hope for a new experience was possible. I realised that her own future had become one of a feeling that this is how it is, and she will forever be looking after her mother. I could see however, that it was possible that she could have a different future, one in which she is free of her mother's neediness, and free of guilt for wanting a life of her own. As we continued in the following sessions to work with these experiences in the past, she also described how hopeless she felt and that the future looked bleak and uninviting.

My own behaviour at the time was that I would demonstrate that I would not hold her captive to my needs, and the corrective emotional experience often involved her doing stuff in the therapy room that allowed for her needs to be placed first. For example, when it was a hot day she wanted the air con on higher than I preferred, and plucked up the courage to ask me that the air con be set at a temperature that she wanted. Another example was when the light overhead bothered her, and she asked for the side light to be turned on. We would discuss these kinds of experiences with me and how they contradicted her preconceived relational assumptions of what to expect. These experiences in therapy also shifted her own fantasies of what could be: that it was possible her needs could be met. With several experiences of a corrected, contradictory experiences, she could, as a result, begin to imagine a different future, one in which she could have her needs me, and I would not be controlling mother.

This working through of the transference but the offering of a corrective experience facilitated her sense of self as being valuable and of having her needs met, however she continued to feel guilt for wanting to leave home, even though, when I asked her what she would want for herself in this regard, she replied she wanted to go but felt it was just a fantasy. This was my clue: that she wished for and verbalised a different future but could not imagine or see it for herself. It was at this time that I could 'see a different future' for her even though she could not see it herself.

In the subsequent sessions, I began to use the potential space of therapy to tentative explore a different future and to ask if she could hope for and imagine things as being different for herself. This invitation to imagine and hope for a different future is done with tender and sensitive care, open to the possibility that my vision of her future may be wrong. I am always guided by her 'talk' of a hoped for future. Using potential space in this regard becomes essential because the 'yet to be formed space' between the two of us became centred on 'what can be' or the 'yet to be future.' Imagining something different in the future, or visioning the future as not a repetition of the past (transference) means that the present-time is one of hope, a hope for a new future. If Marilyn could hope for, and imagine, a different future, of leaving home and not feeling guilty, this would open up a possibility that she could also see herself as leaving. As we talked more about her hopes, and what it would mean for her own future, we also worked with her guilt which was changing. I could see new aspects of her develop, an assertiveness and a new sense of self emerge as she made plans to leave home. It was as if she was becoming a new person as she continued to value her own needs.

Conclusion

As indicated, the capacity to use potential space and have a vision of the future is essential to the process of healing. Patients may not see this future but it is important that the analyst does. The analytic process is partly about the analyst's envisioning a future that is not yet known to the patient, but is only hinted at by the patient. Using potential space creates a possibility for imagination and for what can be. Thus asking the patient to imagine something different is asking the patient to imagine what can be in the future. The experience of the future in psychoanalysis is therefore the process of creating new possibilities, and with it, new ways of relating and being. At one point, Marilyn said to me, which illustrates this vision of a future, "I'll be leaving therapy soon and I don't feel bad about that, I don't feel I am leaving you alone." With that, Marilyn did eventually leave town with her boyfriend and began a new life in a new city.

Finally, Freud first noticed in his work with patients that there was an unconscious tendency to repeat the past in the present. He termed this pattern of repeating the 'repetition compulsion,' and this became the core component of the concept of transference. The phenomenological experience of repeating the past in the present has implications for how the present is experienced and what is possible in the future. Using the potential space of the therapeutic encounter and facilitating a corrective emotional experience allows for a future to be grasped which is important in terms of healing and moving foreword. Without a future, the present is an endless repetition of the past in which there is nothing new, as in the Nietzsche quote above - 'even this spider and this moonlight between the trees.'

REFERENCES

Alexander, F., and French, T. (1946). *Psychoanalytic therapy: Principles and applications.* New York, NY: Ronald Press.

Aron, L. (1997). *A meeting of minds: Mutuality in psychoanalysis*. Hillsdale, NJ: The Analytic Press.

Benjamin, J. (2005). Creating and intersubjective reality. Commentary on a paper by Arnold Rothstein. *Psychoanalytic Dialogues*, 15, 447-457.

Bollas, C. (1989). Forces of destiny. London, UK: Free Association Books.

Cooper, S. (2000). *Objects of hope.* Hillsdale, NJ: The Analytical Press.

Cooper, S. (2004). State of the hope: The new bad object in the therapeutic action of psychoanalysis. *Psychoanalytic Dialogues*, 14(5), 527-551.

Heidegger, M. (1926). *Being and time*. New York: Harper and Row.

Husserl, E. (1904). *The phenomenology of internal time consciousness.* Bloomington, IN: Indiana University Press.

Freud, S. (1896). Further remarks on the neuro-psychoses of defence. In: J. Strachey (Ed. and Trans.), *The standard Edition of the complete psychological works of Sigmund Freud*, Vol. 7, (pp. 116-127). London: Hogarth Press.

Freud, S. (1908), Hysterical phantasies and their relation to bisexuality In: J. Strachey (Ed. and Trans.), *The standard edition of the complete psychological works of Sigmund Freud*, Vol. 9, 155-166. London: Hogarth Press.

Freud, S. (1914). Remembering, repeating and working-through. In: J. Strachey (Ed. and Trans.), *The standard edition of the complete psychological works of Sigmund Freud*, Vol. 12, (pp. 147-156). London: Hogarth Press.

Freud, S. (1915a). Repression. In: J. Strachey (Ed. and Trans.), *The standard edition of the complete psychological works of Sigmund Freud*, Vol. 14, (pp. 141-158). London: Hogarth Press.

Freud, S. (1915b). The unconscious. In: J. Strachey (Ed. and Trans.), *The standard edition of the complete psychological works of Sigmund Freud,* Vol. 14, (pp. 161-216). London: Hogarth Press.

Freud, S. (1920). Beyond the pleasure principle. In: J. Strachey (Ed. and Trans.), *The standard edition of the complete psychological works of Sigmund Freud*, Vol. 18, (pp. 7-64). London, UK: Hogarth Press.

Freud, S. (1966d). Psychotherapy of hysteria from studies on hysteria. In: J. Strachey (Ed. and Trans.), *The standard edition of the complete psychological works of Sigmund Freud*, Vol. 2, (pp. 253-305). London: Hogarth Press (Original work published in 1893).

Kernberg, O. F. (1975). *Borderline conditions and pathological narcissism.* New York, NY: Aronson.

Klein M (1955). *Envy and gratitude and other works*. New York, NY: Delacorte.

Kohut, H. (1977). *The restoration of the self.* New York, NY: International Universities Press.

Kohut, H. (1984). *How does analysis cure*? Chicago: The University of Chicago Press.

Levenson, H. (2010). *Brief dynamic therapy*. Washington, DC: American Psychological Association.

Loewald, H. (1972). The experience of time. In *Papers in psychoanalysis* (pp. 138-148). New Haven: CT, Yale University Press.

Mitchell, S.A. (1993). *Hope and dread in psychoanalysis*. New York: Basic Books.

Mitchell, S. (2000). *Relationality: From attachment to intersubjectivity.* Hillsdale, NJ: The Analytic Press.

Nietzsche, F. (1882/1974). *The gay science* (W. Kaufmann, Trans.). New York, NY: Vintage Books (Original work published 1882).

Searles, H. (1979). *Countertransference and Related Subjects.* Madison, CT: International Universities Press.

Summers, F. (2000). The analyst's vision of the patient and therapeutic action. *Psychoanalytic Psychology*, 17 (3), 547-564.

Summers, F. (2005). *Self creation: Psychoanalytic therapy and the art of the possible.* Hillsdale, NJ: The Analytic Press.

Summers, F. (2007). When one and one makes one. Well, almost. *Contemporary Psychoanalysis*, 43, 638-665.

Summers, F. (2012). Creating new ways of being and relating. *Psychoanalytic dialogues*, 22, 143-161.

Sullivan, H. S. (1953). *The interpersonal theory of psychiatry.* New York, NY: Norton.

Winnicott, D.W. (1951). Transitional objects and transitional phenomena. In: *Through paediatrics to psychoanalysis* (pp. 229-242). New York: Basic Books.

Winnicott, D. (1965). Theory of the parent-infant relationship. In: *Maturational processes and the facilitating environment* (pp. 37-55). New York, NY: International Universities Press.

This work is based upon research supported by the National Research Foundation, South Africa. Any opinion, findings and conclusions or recommendations expressed in this material are those of the author(s) and therefore the NRF do not accept any liability in regard thereto.

nothing" (Freud, 1937, p. 243). For a detailed discussion of Davanloo's view of "super-ego resistance" see Davanloo's papers on the "Clinical Manifestations of Super-ego Pathology" (Davanloo, 1990a,b).

Davanloo picked up where Freud left off. He began to experiment with short-term dynamic techniques in the 1960's. Like others at that time, notably Franz Alexander, Peter Sifneos, David Malan and James Mann, Davanloo initially restricted his short term approach to highly responsive patients with high motivation to change, low resistance and a comparatively simple or even single psychotherapeutic focus (Davanloo, 1975, 1976, 1977, 1978, 1980a,b). This initial work was anchored in psychoanalytic principles and heavily relied on interpretation as a therapeutic factor. However, Davanloo recognized that by utilizing such strict selection (and thereby exclusion) criteria he could only effectively treat a small percentage of patients who presented for treatment.

In the 1970's, not satisfied with "bowing" to the superior destructive forces in the unconscious, Davanloo began to focus on highly resistant patients with severe phobic and obsessional neuroses, and syntonic character pathology (Davanloo, 1979a) with the aim of increasing the range of patients who could be treated. By the use of audio-visual recording, he painstakingly reviewed his work and refined his interventions, culminating in the technique of "Total Removal of Resistance" in a single interview. With removal of resistance, the direct experience of transference feelings was mobilized and led to an immediate and clear view of the psychopathological dynamic forces in the patient's unconscious that were responsible for the symptom and characterological disturbances. This was the beginning of his technique of Intensive Short-Term Dynamic Psychotherapy (Davanloo, 1975, 1977, 1984). Based on patients' own description of this process he called this technique "Unlocking the Unconscious" (Davanloo, 1990e,f).

In the 1980's Davanloo further expanded the spectrum of patients who could be successfully treated with Intensive Short-term Dynamic Psychotherapy, to include those with depressive disorders, somatization and functional disorders, and panic disorder. Many of these cases have been published (Davanloo, 1978; 1979a; 1980a; 1990a,b, c, d, e, f, g, h). Continuing in the 80's and early 90's he focused on the application of the technique to a spectrum of patients with fragile and borderline character structure. Many of these cases were presented in a number of international symposia (Davanloo, 1993a,b, 1998).

In the later 1990s he refined his technique and interventions further, focusing on what he called the highly powerful method of "Mobilization of the Unconscious." His focus was on the application of this method to extremely resistant patients with the most the complex pathogenic unconscious. He further refined his technique of rapid mobilization of tactical and characterologic defenses (Davanloo, 2000d,e), "crystallization" of the resistance in the transference, rapid activation of the transference component of the resistance and the complex transference feelings, mobilization of the "Unconscious Therapeutic Alliance," direct access to the psychopathological dynamic forces, and "Multidimensional Unconscious Structural Changes." (Davanloo, 1998, 2013, 2014).

He continued this work into the 2000's primarily in the form of training workshops in North America and Europe, utilizing live closed circuit audio-visual observation and supervision. In 2007 he instituted the Montreal Training Workshops in Mobilization of the Unconscious (Davanloo, 2007-2016) to which I had the privilege of attending through 2014. Audio-visually recorded vignettes from this program have been presented in Montreal in the ongoing annual audio-visual symposia (Davanloo, 2007-2015). During this period Davanloo developed and refined his understanding of the role of "Fusion" of primitive murderous rage, unconscious guilt, and sexual feeling in the unconscious. It is this Fusion that is the "pathogenic destructive dynamic system in the unconscious." Other terms he has employed for this destructive system are "Major Resistance," the "Destructive Organization of the Unconscious," the masochistic resistance of the superego (Davanloo 1990a,b), and the "Perpetrator of the Unconscious" (Davanloo, 2000a, 2001; Beeber, 1999a,bc,). The rapid removal of this destructive force in the unconscious is the central task of the therapist in these techniques (Davanloo, 2011) and distinguishes Davanloo's Intensive Short-term Dynamic Psychotherapy and Mobilization of the Unconscious from other techniques of short-term therapy.

For the past several years, Davanloo has placed major emphasis on the identification and removal of Transference Neurosis as a central factor complicating, if not preventing, the removal of the original fusion in the unconscious. This has been the focus of many of the training workshops since 2009. The programs of training in the Mobilization of the Unconscious, Multidimensional Unconscious Structural Change, and Transference Neurosis have been described in detail in numerous presentations at symposia under the direction of Davanloo, over the past several years (Davanloo, 2007-2016).

In this chapter I will present the basic principles that serve as a foundation of Davanloo's metapsychology and psychotherapeutic techniques.

SPECTRUM OF PSYCHOPATHOLOGY

In his systematic work in the 70's and 80's he demonstrated that the technique of Davanloo's Intensive Short-term Dynamic Psychotherapy (DISTDP) could create multidimensional unconscious structural changes in a wide range of patients (Davanloo, 2000a). He initially described two broad groups of patients that were treatable with DISTDP, (1) a spectrum of psychoneurotic patients, and (2) a spectrum of patients with fragile character structure (Davanloo, 2005 pp.2650-2651). Patients with severely fragile character structure have an extremely low capacity to tolerate anxiety and painful affects. They easily become flooded with anxiety, with consequent disruption of cognitive and perceptual functions. They have access to primitive defenses such as projection, projective identification, and explosive discharge of affect and temper tantrums and are therefore usually excluded from short-term dynamic psychotherapies. Davanloo has shown that they *can* be treated with DISTDP, but that they cannot withstand the impact of their unconscious in a single interview. They require a phase, sometimes a quite extended phase, of multidimensional unconscious structural changes (MDUSC), raising the capacity to tolerate anxiety and painful feelings, and bringing changes to the defensive structure, before the patient can access their unconscious (Davanloo, 2005 p.2651). Davanloo has presented this important process of MDUSC in detail in recent symposia (Davanloo, 2012, 2013) and this topic requires much further discussion. The process of MDUSC underlies all of Davanloo's techniques and methods.

The "Spectrum of Psychoneurotic Disorders" represents the range of patients for whom Davanloo has demonstrated that access to the core neurotic structure can be achieved in a single session via the technique of "Total Removal of the Resistance." (Figure 1).

For a detailed discussion of the diagnostic spectrum see Davanloo's article on this topic (Davanloo, 2000a). Briefly on the left side of the spectrum patients are highly responsive, highly motivated and show low resistance. They have a high capacity to tolerate anxiety and painful affects. They have circumscribed problems, often only a single psychotherapeutic focus. There is an absence of early trauma and unconscious guilt, and the course of treatment is generally quite short. Davanloo reports treatment in a single session (Davanloo, 2000a). This type of patient is quite rare in the typical psychotherapeutic practice. On the mid-left of the spectrum patients have a moderate degree of resistance and symptoms are more diffuse. Character pathology is present to some degree but is often dystonic. Trauma is usually present but generally occurs after the age of 4 or 5. There is unconscious violent rage and guilt- and grief-laden feelings in the unconscious in relation to early figures. As one moves further rightward, resistance is higher, symptom disturbances become more diffuse, and characterological disturbances become more diffuse, complex and generally syntonic. Masochistic character traits become manifest. Trauma occurs earlier, and is more intense. Unconscious rage takes on a murderous quality. Guilt and grief-laden unconscious feelings become more intense. On the far right side, resistance is at its highest, symptom and character disturbances are quite diffuse and complex; and there is a high degree of masochism present. Trauma is often early, (often in the first one to three years of life), and can be quite severe and repetitive. Unconscious rage has a primitive quality and often involves torturous feelings; sexualized feelings become fused with rage. Guilt and grief-laden feelings are extremely intense. This constellation of early trauma, pain of trauma, unconscious primitive torturous or murderous rage, intense guilt and grief-laden feelings and masochism in the character structure is what Davanloo termed "The Perpetrator of the Unconscious" (Davanloo, 1990a, 2001, p.28; Beeber, 1999a, b, c).

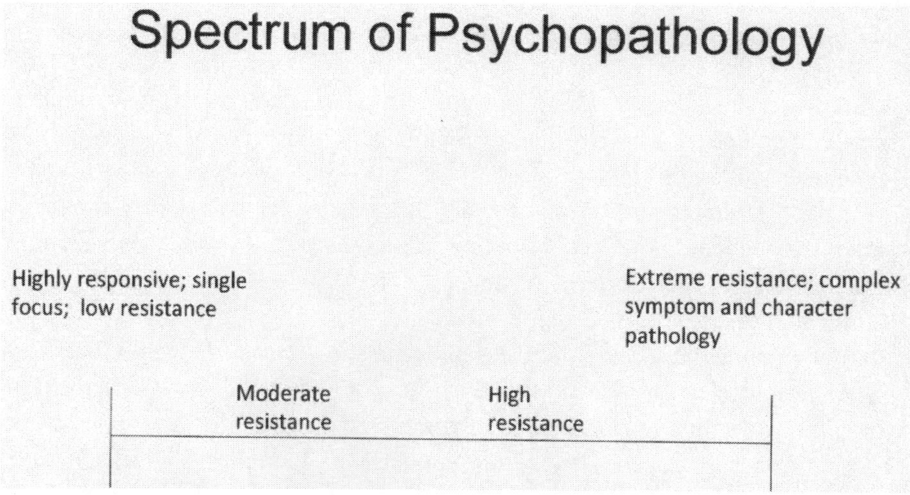

Figure 1. Spectrum of Psychoneurotic Disorders (adapted from Davanloo, 2000a. Used with permission of the author).

PSYCHOPATHOLOGICAL DYNAMIC FORCES

Based on his observations and systematic review of audio-visually recorded case series over the decades of his clinical research, Davanloo elicited and described the Psychopathological Dynamic Forces at work in human neurosis. They are represented schematically as a series of concentric layers in the Unconscious (Davanloo, 2000c, p. 102) (Figure 2).

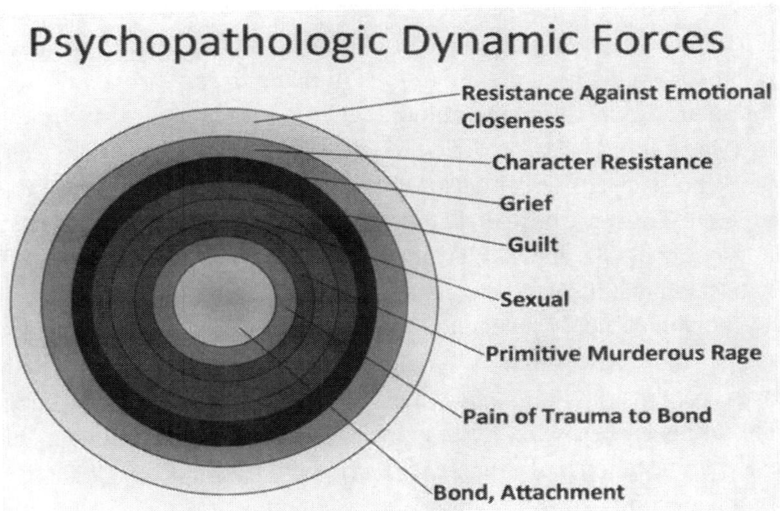

Figure 2. Psychopathologic Dynamic Forces (adapted from Davanloo, 2000c, p. 102. Used with permission of the author).

At the center of these forces is the bond and attachment to the early parental figures. For patients on the right side of the spectrum this bond is traumatized and the trauma is experienced as extremely painful. In reaction to the trauma and pain of trauma, is rage directed at the attachment figure. This rage is qualitatively and quantitatively in proportion to the trauma. While constitutional factors may play a role, generally the more intense and repetitive the trauma, the more intense is the reactive rage. As one moves rightward on the spectrum of psychoneurotic disturbance the rage takes on a murderous, primitive murderous, and primitive torturous/murderous quality. Unconscious guilt results in reaction to the rage (that has been directed at the attachment figure who has been loved as well) and it too, is in proportion to the intensity of the trauma and rage. This unconscious guilt is a highly pathogenic system which is the dynamic engine to the need for self-sabotage and self-punishment, i.e., masochism in the character. As the rage may have a murderous quality, there is also grief-laden unconscious feeling in reaction to the loss (murder) of the early parental figure. Actual early losses may also give further rise to Grief-laden unconscious feelings.

These unconscious feelings are not experienced separately and remain in a "fused" state in the unconscious, defended against by the development of characterologic defenses (character resistances). In addition, Davanloo uniquely observed and described a specific constellation of character defenses whose aim is to defend against reactivating the early attachment and traumatic painful feelings by fending off closeness and intimacy in current interpersonal relationships. He identified these defenses in many of his early cases, notably the "German Architect" (Davanloo, 1990i, p.14), the "Machine Gun Woman"(Davanloo, 1990c, pp. 62,64,68,74; 1990b, pp. 209,214, 218.) and the "Woman Who Bruised Her Thigh" (Davanloo, 1990e, p. 119). In the "Case of the Corporate Lawyer" he called this constellation of defenses "Resistance Against Emotional Closeness" (Davanloo, 1990f, pp.132, 134-136,156).

Unconscious Guilt plays the central role in Davanloo's understanding of the Psychopathological Dynamic Forces. He uses the terms "Major Resistance" and "Resistance of Guilt" synonymously, both of which are present in patients in the middle and on the ride side of the diagnostic spectrum. In his earlier work, he described the effects of unconscious Guilt as "clinical manifestations of Superego Pathology (Davanloo, 1990a,b)." He later, in referring to the entire constellation of attachment/trauma, abandonment in the early phase of life/murderous rage/intense guilt- and grief-laden unconscious feeling/masochism in the character, coined the term "Perpetrator of the Unconscious." (Davanloo, 2000a, p.4).

More recently he has adopted the term "Fusion" to describe this dynamic constellation in the unconscious. The Major Resistance of Guilt does not allow the pain of the trauma, the reactive rage and sexualized feeling to be experienced as separate feelings. Instead these feelings are bound together in the unconscious - as if they were set in concrete and are inaccessible (Represented schematically in Figure 3).

He called the "Fusion of Guilt and Primitive Murderous Rage" (as well as the other feelings) "a pathogenic destructive dynamic system in the unconscious (Davanloo, 2009, 2010, 2011). A major task of the therapist is "the rapid removal of this destructive system" (Davanloo, 2009, 2010, 2011). It is only through removal of Fusion, that the dynamic forces of the Original Neurosis become accessible. He went on further to state that the age of the trauma was critical and that patients traumatized at an early age, for whom fusion takes place at age 3 or earlier have far more complexity in their unconscious, than those for whom the trauma and fusion takes place at age 4 or older. This complexity arising from early fusion requires a more extensive process of Mobilization of the Unconscious and of Multidimensional Unconscious Structural Change before a more traditional course of DISTDP can be initiated. In contrast, patients whose fusion takes place at age 4 or later can be treated in a much more straightforward fashion with DISTDP (Davanloo, 2013, 2014). The complexities of Multidimensional Unconscious Structural Change go beyond the scope of this introductory chapter and require much further discussion.

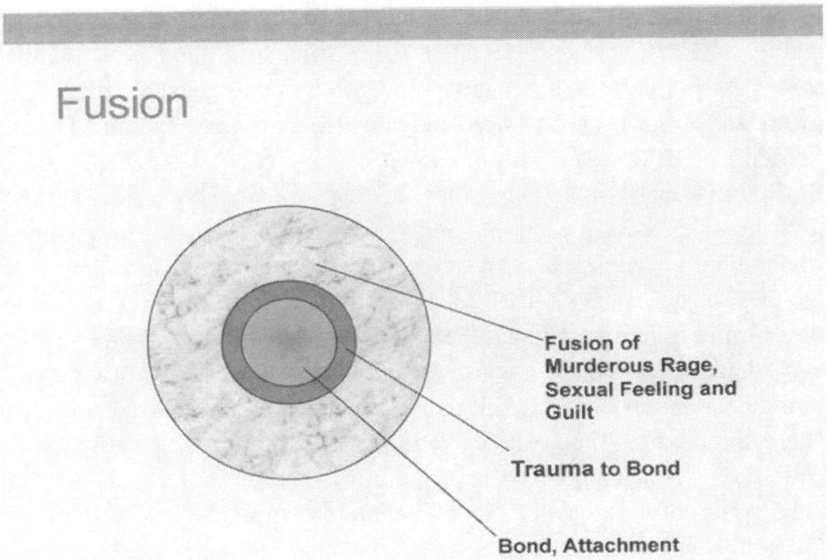

Figure 3. Fusion of Primitive Murderous Rage and Guilt (adapted from Davanloo, 2009. Used with permission of the author).

Triangle of Persons and Triangle of Conflict: Historical Perspective

The constellation of intense, conflictual feelings described above remains fused in the Unconscious as a result of the Major Resistance. When issues in current life and current relationships reverberate emotionally with these feelings from the past, unconscious anxiety is mobilized. Anxiety in turn mobilizes characterologic defenses, which may or may not be adequate to manage the anxiety. If not, more malignant character defenses may be mobilized or the person may become symptomatic with anxiety and its concomitants. These basic principles of Impulse/Anxiety/Defense and the relationship of Current Life/ Past/ Therapeutic Relationship (Transference) are cornerstones of most psychodynamic theory (Fenichel, 1945; Greenson, 1967).

These concepts have been represented schematically by a number of analytic theorists. Menninger coined the term "Triangle of Insight" (Menninger 1958). He felt that the insight necessary for successful psychoanalysis rested on the recognition of the relationship of the past, current life and the analytic situation.

"In the proper sense of the word and in the useful sense for psychoanalytic technique, insight is the simultaneous identification of the characteristic behavior pattern in all three situations, together with an understanding of why they were and are used as they were and are." (Menninger, 1958, p. 148).

Ezriel, (1959,1992) writing about the role of transference in psychoanalysis and in group therapies also described the triangular relationship of the past, present life and the transference relationship. He noted that the patient is "consciously or unconsciously attempting, to establish with me in that session one kind of relationship which he requires ("required" relationship) in order to avoid another (the "avoided" relationship), because he believes that this second relationship would inevitably lead to a third, the "calamitous" relationship." He felt that by interpreting these three elements in the "here and now" of the analytic situation or therapy group, "reality testing" was induced which would lead to symptom reduction and character change (Ezriel's notion of the so called "mutative interpretation").

In both these systems interpretation is the central therapeutic intervention. The therapist notes and points out over the course of therapy the patterns of issues in (1) current relationships; (2) the transference patterns of behavior; and (3) relationships in the past, primarily with family members. Links are drawn between Transference, Current and Past.

In the mid-70's Davanloo presented his pioneering work, along with Malan, Sifneos, Marmor and others, in the for of the First and Second International Symposia and Workshops on Short-Term Dynamic Psychotherapy (Davanloo, 1975,1976). As a result of the success of these two symposia, Davanloo set up the Third International Symposia and Workshops in 1977 and founded the Institute of Short-Term Dynamic Psychotherapy at Montreal General Hospital and McGill University (Davanloo, 1977, 1980a p. ix). It was at these symposia that he presented his method of Short-Term

Dynamic Psychotherapy accompanied by audio-visually recorded actual sessions with patients. His book, *Short-Term Dynamic Psychotherapy* grew out of these symposia (Davanloo, 1980a). It was here that he published his method (Davanloo, 1980b), which at this point in time still relied on the use of interpretation. His method is elaborated in other publications of his at that time as well (Davanloo, 1978; 1979b).

In this early phase of his work Davanloo's method focused on understanding and clarifying for the patient the relationship of Impulses and Feelings (I/F), Anxiety (A) and Defense (D) in the Past (P), the Current Life of the patient (C) and in the Transference (T) (Davanloo 1980a p.52, pp.81-82). He, like others at the time, believed that it was the interpretation of the T-C-P link, accompanied by insight into the relationship of Impulse/Feeling to Anxiety to Defense that were the main psychotherapeutic factors (Davanloo 1980a p.91). I include this process of interpretation of I/F-A-D and the T-C-P link for its historical place in the development of Davanloo's Metapsychology of the Unconscious. He later came to the conclusion that that interpretation was ineffective as a major therapeutic factor and abandoned interpretation entirely as a therapeutic technique. By virtue of his systematic review of his audio-visual recordings he came to see the serious limitations of the process of interpretation. This motivated him to refine his interventions and develop his further understanding of the metapsychology of the unconscious. His current focus on his techniques of Mobilization of the Unconscious and Total Removal of Resistance and Multidimensional Unconscious Structural Change (Davanloo, 2007-2015) go far beyond interpretation of the psychoanalytic triangles.

Beyond the Triangle of Conflict

Davanloo took the basic analytic concepts of the relationship of impulse/feelings to anxiety and defense –the triangle of conflict- much further. He noted that neurotic patients have great difficulty distinguishing feeling from anxiety from defense. He also observed that there was much confusion among psychotherapists as well about what constituted a feeling or a defense, and what distinguished one feeling from another. This is especially true of the painful affect-laden feelings of guilt and grief. As a result of his systematic clinical research with a wide variety of patients, Davanloo observed and described straightforward guidelines for distinguishing impulse/feeling from anxiety and defense, based on their psychophysiological concomitants.

PSYCHOPHYSIOLOGICAL CONCOMITANTS OF FEELINGS

On Davanloo's view "feelings" have psychophysiological concomitants. "I feel angry" may be merely a statement of thought, a purely cognitive experience with no physiological concomitant, and may therefore serve a defensive function. He called this type of resistance a "tactical defense" (Davanloo 2000d,e). Only if one were to focus on *how* the person actually *experiences* the "anger" can one tell if this is a true feeling or merely a defense. Taking the feelings one at a time, Davanloo describes clear physiologic concomitants as the basis for each.

Rage, murderous rage, and torturous murderous rage all involve the mobilization of a specific system, which Davanloo calls the Neurobiological or Somatic Pathway (NBP) of Murderous Rage. Patients describe this experience as a force of energy, often hot, like a "fireball" or "volcano" that starts in the pelvis or lower abdomen, then moves upward into the chest, where it moves up and down for a brief period of time, and then moves up towards the head. It then feels as if it were moving into the arms, to the hands, accompanied by the impulse to grab the other person. (Davanloo, 2001 p.40). This *internal* experience, which is not associated with *external* acting on the rage, stands in contrast to " explosive discharge of affect," a defense mechanism associated with activity such as yelling or punching walls in the form of a temper tantrum. This latter explosive discharge is considered a regressive defense against the *actual experience* of unconscious murderous rage (Davanloo, 2005 p.2652). Hence, rageful feeling is here distinguished from angry thought and regressive defense.

Guilt is experienced as a wave of deeply painful feeling starting in the chest and involving the upper airway, bronchi, pharynx and larynx. It is experienced in sharp waves of high intensity and may be associated with gasping or sharp, painful sobbing. In contrast, Grief-laden feelings are also painful waves in the chest and but involve the lower airway. The upper airway and pharynx are generally not involved. Waves are smoother and of lower amplitude. Sobbing is also smoother and the entire feeling is less painful than the pain of Guilt (Davanloo, 2001 pp.44-45). In contrast, weepiness, (often having a whining quality), is a regressive defense against murderous rage and, like explosive discharge, acts like the opening of a valve on a pressure cooker to reduce the buildup of unconscious anxiety that had been mobilized by the rage. The person is unlikely to be able to identify the origin of the tears and not associate it with any particular painful memory or particular issue.

However, if the person is then asked what it is that they are experiencing they describe anxiety (Davanloo, 1990c, p.64-67).

Sexual feeling has obvious physiologic concomitants as well. In women there is tumescence of the nipples and clitoris as well as lubrication of the vagina. In men there is erection of the penis. (Davanloo 1990j, 1991, 1993a,b). Without these physiologic concomitants of "feelings" being present one is likely dealing with tactical defenses despite the fact that the patient uses the word "feeling." This simple sounding principle is not widely understood. It is extremely important to note that when there is Fusion in the unconscious, the person has great difficulty being in touch with his/her "feelings." It is only when Fusion is removed, that unconscious "feeling" can actually be experienced fully and consciously (Davanloo, 2005 p.2647, 2009-2014).

Discharge Pattern of Unconscious Anxiety

Another of Davanloo's unique and elegant observations involves the psychophysiological discharge pattern of unconscious anxiety. He noted that for some patients, unconscious anxiety is primarily manifested in the form of tension in the voluntary (striated musculature. The voluntary muscles provide a huge reservoir for anxiety and thus these patients show a relatively high capacity to tolerate anxiety (and the underlying unconscious feelings) (Davanloo, 1990j, 1991, 1993a, 2005, p.2637). In the initial interview with these patients, Davanloo observed the progression of the mobilization of unconscious anxiety in the striated muscle system. He noted that anxiety in the form of muscle tension is often initially seen as tension in the hands, thumbs and fingers. As it increases in intensity it involves the pronator and supinator muscles of the forearm, leading to a squeezing movement of the hands. Tension increases up the arms to the neck, with tension in the sternocleidomastoids, and muscles of the jaw. Higher anxiety creates tension in the intercostal and sub diaphragmatic muscles leading to tightness in the chest wall and sighing respirations. (Davanloo, 2005, p.2642). Some patients however, have very little access to striated muscle tension when anxious. Instead anxiety is channeled primarily into the autonomic nervous system (smooth muscle). In this situation, capacity to tolerate anxiety is much lower and patients become symptomatic with autonomic manifestations such as sweating, rapid heart and shallow breathing, queasy stomach, nausea, vomiting, abdominal cramping, diarrhea, or bronchospasm and experience muscular weakness rather than tension. (Davanloo, 2005, p.2642). The third group of patients also lacks access to the striated muscle discharge pattern of anxiety. Instead anxiety is channeled into the cognitive and perceptual system. These patients have an extremely low capacity to tolerate anxiety. They easily become flooded with anxiety and develop cognitive and perceptual disturbances such as drifting of their thoughts, light-headedness, visual blurring, disrupted thoughts, fainting, and even micro psychotic symptoms such as brief periods of auditory illusions or hallucinations, and mild paranoid ideas. (Davanloo, 1993a,b). These observations have major significance for the application of Davanloo's technique of mobilizing the unconscious. Patients with access to striated muscle tension have the capacity to withstand the feelings in their unconscious and the anxiety it activates; and one can access the unconscious in a single session (Davanloo, 2001.) For patients with predominantly autonomic discharge, a more graded and step-wise approach is necessary. This can be done in one extended session or in a few sessions, until such time as structural change has been accomplished in the discharge pattern from the autonomic system to striated muscle tension. (Davanloo, 1990g,h; Whittemore 1998). For patients with primarily cognitive and perceptual discharge of anxiety, a period of several sessions (sometimes in the range of 10-20 sessions or more) is necessary to bring unconscious structural change at the dimensions of (1) increased capacity to tolerate anxiety, (2) discharge into striated musculature, (3) increased capacity to tolerate rage, (4) increased capacity to tolerate painful feelings, (5) changes in the defensive organization from more primitive defenses (for example projection and projective identification) to more obsessional defenses. Once these multidimensional unconscious structural changes have been accomplished, the patient can now withstand the impact of his/her unconscious (Davanloo, 2005, p.2642, 1993a,b). It is extremely important in the first phase of the initial interview to determine the degree of the patient's anxiety and its discharge pattern as well as the patient's capacity to tolerate anxiety (Davanloo, 1990j, 1991, 1993a,b).

Unconscious Defensive System

Davanloo observed, in a wide range of patients, a complex defensive system, which needs to be recognized and understood by any practitioner hoping to treat the full spectrum of patients with DISTDP or any other dynamic technique for that matter. Each patient's defensive structure is unique and most be actively and rapidly detected and mobilized if one wants to achieve "Total Removal of Resistance" in a single or even a few sessions.

Most dynamic therapists are familiar with characterologic defenses. Many have been elucidated by Wilhelm Reich (1933/1980). Very few therapists are familiar, however, with what Davanloo refers to as "Tactical Defenses" (Davanloo, 2000d,e). These defenses are unconscious maneuvers on the part of the patient to reduce anxiety and avoid uncomfortable feelings. The person's responses seem to answer a question from the therapist or seem to provide a fruitful direction for the interview but are actually tactics geared towards managing anxiety and blocking the further mobilization of feelings. Typical tactical defenses in the early phase of the interview include: diverting to the past, generalizing, using a word of lower intensity to cover the intensity of a feeling and minimization. These defenses may be used alone or in combination. A brief example will suffice. When asked how he feels towards the therapist, the patient, sitting forward, hands tightly clasped, scowling, responds, "I guess maybe I felt a little bit irritated," a quintuple tactical defense against a negative feeling. One can apply pressure to the underlying feeling by blocking the tactical defense with specific targeted interventions. For example, at the beginning of the first interview a patient is asked what are the difficulties he's experiencing for which he wants help. The patient replies, "Well my father died when I was a 5 years old." While this is likely important, it does not really answer the therapists' question. Viewing this response as a the tactical defense of diverting to the distant past, the therapist responds, "Oh, I see. We can get to that. But what are the current difficulties you are having, that you decided to come now for my help." This intervention blocks the defense of diverting. The patient clasps his hands together, looks away from the therapist and responds, "I was abusing alcohol until two years ago…" to which the therapist replies, "So what are the current difficulties…" The patient now shifts in the chair, puts his hands on top of his head, sighs deeply and says "I suffer from anxiety." More anxiety is mobilized by the intervention in the form of increasing striated muscle tension and new tactical defense is mobilized. This increase in striated muscle tension confirms the therapist's view that he/she is encountering tactical defense and is a green light to increase the pressure on the defensive system. The ability to recognize tactical defenses and respond accordingly is an essential feature of Davanloo's techniques (Davanloo, 2000d,e).

Another of Davanloo's unique contributions is his observation of a specific set of characterologic defenses that are geared towards defending against intimacy and closeness – what he calls "Resistance Against Emotional Closeness." By avoiding and resisting closeness, one tries to prevent activation of the feelings that are at the core of the neurosis, namely attachment, bond, love, trauma, pain of trauma, and the reactive rage and guilt associated with the trauma. Resistance Against Emotional Closeness takes many forms and is a major emphasis in all of Davanloo's techniques. It is through recognition and systematic work on this constellation of defenses in the Transference that Davanloo achieves the mobilization of the unconscious necessary for access to the psychopathological destructive dynamic forces (Davanloo, 2005 pp. 2637-2638).

Yet another contribution is Davanloo's recognition of the importance of the mobilization of the Transference Component of the Resistance. Any resistant patient enters the interview in a divided state. Though the patient wants the therapist's help, they also want to reduce anxiety and at the same time avoid rageful and painful feelings. Initially the patient employs their typical characterologic defenses but as the therapist keeps up the pressure by blocking the defenses the defenses "tilt" towards the therapist. That is, the more the therapist blocks the avoiding, the harder the patient tries to distance and keep the therapist out of their intimate thoughts and intimate feelings. This occurs at the same time the patient recognizes that they need and want the therapist's help. Not just resisting anyone now, the patient is actively resisting the efforts of the therapist to help them despite the patient's wish to cooperate and collaborate with the therapist. This creates an intrapsychic tension within the patient, between the resistance and the transference and activates what Davanloo terms the Transference Component of the Resistance (TCR) and concomitant Complex Transference Feelings (CTF). It is the very mobilization of the TCR and the CTF that leads to an intrapsychic crisis, and ultimately to access to the core neurotic structure (Davanloo, 2005 p.2630; 2007-15).

Still other defenses are in the category of regressive defenses such as weepiness or explosive discharge of affect, which are attempts to reduce anxiety, and defend against the experience of (murderous) rage. They should not be confused with the actual experience of rage (Davanloo, 1987/1990c, pp.64-67; 2005 p. 2652).

Lastly is the category of what Davanloo refers to as malignant character defenses, such as projection, projective identification, defiance (often "wrapped in a bouquet of seeming compliance"), oppositional character traits, and accusation, to name a few (Davanloo, 2007-15). This last category of defense often indicates impairment in the defensive system, which is characteristic of those with Fusion in the first three years of life.

MOBILIZATION OF THE UNCONSCIOUS

Mobilization of the Unconscious refers to both an overarching aim and principle of Davanloo's techniques, and to a specific teaching and learning process Davanloo uses in a specific form of workshop for the training of DISTDP therapists. In the first sense, Mobilization of the Unconscious is the process by which the therapist activates the patient's unconscious in an attempt to bring all of the Psychopathological Dynamic Forces to consciousness so that they are available to the patient and therapist to be worked through via the processes of Psychoanalytic Investigation and Multidimensional Unconscious Structural Change (Davanloo, 2010, 2011, 2014). These latter therapeutic techniques, Psychoanalytic Investigation and Multidimensional Unconscious Structural Change require much more extensive elaboration than can be addressed in this overview.

Briefly, Mobilization of the Unconscious is accomplished by Davanloo's techniques of the application of the Central Dynamic Sequence and Total Removal of the Resistance (described below). The process depends heavily on the twin factors of the Transference Feeling and the Transference Component of the Resistance. As the resistant patient is both trying to cooperate with the therapist and defeat the therapist at the same time, it is through the application of the Central Dynamic Sequence that the therapist rapidly achieves mobilization of the tactical organization of the patient's resistance as well as their characterological defenses. Through the process of relentlessly trying to liberate the patient from the destructive forces in their unconscious and at the same time not being put off by the patient's efforts to delay and defeat the process, there is activation of intense Complex Transference Feeling (CTF). The patient experiences positive feelings and a sense of gratitude towards the therapist for the relentless efforts to help the patient. At the same the patient experiences negative, rageful feelings towards the therapist for not allowing their usual defenses to work. As characterological and tactical defenses fail to thwart the therapist, the resistance redoubles its efforts and becomes tilted in the direction of therapist. The patient is not merely defending and distancing as they do in every relationship, but is now resisting and distancing the therapist, despite it being against their best interests. This leads to crystallization of resistance in the transference and activation of the Transference Component of the Resistance (TCR) (Davanloo, 2005 pp.2630-31). It is at this point that Davanloo brings his most powerful intervention, the Head-On-Collision with the Resistance into operation. Following application of the technique of Head-On-Collision with the Destructive Organization of the Resistance there is de-fusion of the primitive murderous rage and guilt with direct experience of the transference feeling in the here and now of the interview. As a result of the de-fusion, there is mobilization of the Neurobiological Pathway of the Murderous Rage in the Transference. This is accompanied by the mobilization of a new force in the Unconscious, namely the Unconscious Therapeutic Alliance (UTA). A hallmark of "Mobilization" is now achieved, namely the predominance of affective responses over cognitive responses, and the predominance of the UTA over the forces of the Resistance. There is can now be direct access to the psychopathological dynamic forces heretofore having been repressed in the unconscious. The unconscious in now said to be "Unlocked" (Davanloo, 2001 pp.30-46; 2005 pp.2630-2631, 2636-2641).

TECHNIQUE OF TOTAL REMOVAL OF RESISTANCE

Akin to Mobilization is Davanloo's technique of Total Removal of Resistance, which will be briefly reviewed. Patients on the right side of the spectrum are highly resistant and yet access to the core neurotic structure is possible in a single interview. Davanloo has presented this process in many international symposia since the 1970's. A detailed description of the process is found his article "Intensive Short-Term Dynamic Psychotherapy: Extended Major Direct Access to the Unconscious" (Davanloo, 2001). Typically, the interview progresses through a series of phases, which he called the Central Dynamic Sequence (Davanloo, 1990e p. 101; 2001 pp.30-32).

Briefly, the phases of the interview consist of:

(1) Inquiry
(2) Pressure
(3) Challenge
(4) Transference Resistance
    a. Crystallization of the resistance in the transference, the transference component of the resistance
    b. Head on collision with the resistance in the transference, its destructive role and with Resistance Against Emotional Closeness
    c. Mobilization of the Unconscious Therapeutic Alliance against the forces of the resistance
    d. Creation of an intrapsychic crisis, loosening of the psychic system
(5) Direct Access to the Unconscious

(6) Analysis of the Process (Analysis of the Transference) and Consolidation
(7) Psychoanalytic Investigation – a dynamic exploration of the unconscious
(8) Recapitulation, Consolidation and Psychotherapeutic Planning

Essentially, the initial process is one of establishing the psychodynamic diagnosis – i.e., where the patient lies on the psychodiagnostic spectrum, If the patient evidences an intact defensive system with a robust tactical defensive organization, discharge of anxiety in the form of striated muscle tension with a relatively high capacity to tolerate anxiety and no indication of fragility in the character, direct access to the unconscious is indicated. One then can apply the technique of Total Removal of Resistance via application of the Central Dynamic Sequence. The aim of the Phase of Pressure is to mobilize the tactical system of defense and the complex transference feeling (Davanloo, 2000f). As this is accomplished, the unconscious of the patient becomes alarmed and the characterologic and tactical defenses now tilt in the dimension of the therapist to defend against the rising Transference Feelings (CTF). With further pressure, there is now "crystallization" of the resistance in the transference. At this point the therapist can begin to apply passing and then systematic challenge to the resistances in the transference, with further pressure, which gives further rise to the Transference Component of the Resistance (TCR) (Davanloo, 2000g). By challenging the destructiveness of the resistances, pointing out that the defenses have been paralyzing and crippling for the patient, the therapist turns the patient against the resistance, showing no respect for the defenses that have been damaging the patient's life. At the same time the therapist shows the highest respect for the patient, highlighting that the patient has the capacity to change and does not deserve to lead a life of self-sabotage and self-punishment. In part the patient is identified with their defenses and becomes angry with the therapist for not allowing the defenses to work. At the same time the patient recognizes the self-damaging and self-defeating aspects of the resistances and is highly appreciative of the therapists relentless efforts to help free them from this internal perpetrator of destruction. This intrapsychic conflict of mixed feelings leads to further mobilization of the triple factors of Complex Transference Feeling, the Transference Component of the Resistance and the Unconscious Therapeutic Alliance (UTA). The process continues in the phase of Transference Resistance culminating in the application of Davanloo's most powerful intervention, namely the Head on Collision (HOC) with the Resistance

Against Emotional Closeness and with the Destructive Organization of the Resistance (Davanloo, 2000h). By definition, the Head on Collision entails the total blockade of all the forces of the resistance. Consisting of a possible 16 or 17 elements, various components of the Head on Collision may be assembled to form specific interventions in specific situations. As a result of its application, Transference Feeling intensifies greatly and there is a state of palpable tension between the Resistance and the Unconscious Therapeutic Alliance. The patient is exquisitely aware that though they want their utmost, to collaborate and cooperate with the therapist, they are also heavily resisting the therapist's efforts to get to their most intimate thoughts and feelings and to help free the patient from the destructive "master" of unconscious guilt to which they has been a "slave." This creates a major intrapsychic crisis and loosens the whole psychic system as it reverberates with the core of the psychopathological dynamic forces. There is now further activation of the Neurobiological Pathway of Murderous Rage (fusion age 4 or later) or Sadistic Primitive Murderous Rage (fusion age 3 or earlier) (Davanloo, 2007-2014b, 2011, 2012, 2013, 2014.). Patients have described this process as "breaking through" or "unlocking the unconscious." At this point in the interview, there is dominance of the Unconscious Therapeutic Alliance and total removal of resistance. Unconscious anxiety drops and the patient is brought face to face with his/her unconscious. Typically the patient has visual imagery of the murdered body of the therapist and a feeling of sadness begins to emerge. In the process of looking at the body and describing the damage to the therapist, the patient is asked to focus on the visual image of the eyes of the dead body and to describe the expression, communication from the eyes and most importantly the eye color. If the Unconscious Therapeutic Alliance has been sufficiently mobilized what transpires is that the imagery of the therapist's eyes become visually transferred to the eyes of an early figure in the patient's life – usually a parent. At this point the Neurobiological Pathway of Guilt becomes mobilized with the experience of waves of extremely painful Guilt-laden feeling typically lasting from upwards of 8 minutes. This is followed by the experience of positive loving feelings for the parent. Waves of Grief-laden feelings are experienced for the (unconscious) murder of the loved one, for loss of the bond as a result of early trauma, for the murderous feeling and for the lost years in their relationship (Davanloo, 2001, pp.59-62). This then leads to the phase of Analysis of the Process with recapitulation of the session and a Phase of Consolidation (Davanloo, 2001, pp.30, 46,54), followed by a phase of extensive dynamic, psychoanalytic investigation of the patients early years and relationships to the key figures in early life. This exploration is often accompanied by additional breakthroughs of feeling in relation to these figures from the past. There is a major focus here on creating multidimensional unconscious structural changes in the dimensions of anxiety, defense, feeling and memory. The initial session usually ends with a phase of further recapitulation, consolidation, and psychotherapeutic planning (Davanloo, 2001, p. 64).

COURSE OF DISTDP

Generally, the full Spectrum of Psychoneurotic Disorders and the Spectrum of Fragility can be treated with one or another variation of DISTDP. As noted earlier, patients with fragility in their character with an extremely low capacity to tolerate anxiety and painful affects are typically excluded from other forms of short-term dynamic therapy. However, utilizing Davanloo's method of an extensive phase (5-20 sessions duration) of Multidimensional Unconscious Structural Change many of these patients can be then treated with a variation of DISTDP. A full course of treatment can be upwards of 60-80 sessions for patients with fragile character structure though symptomatic improvement can be achieved within the first 20 sessions (Davanloo, 2000a, p.4; 1993a,b; 2005, pp.2650-2651). This obviously is not "short-term" therapy in its usual sense but certainly a much shorter course than that of typical psychodynamic psychotherapy.

Patients with access to autonomic discharge or with characterologic depression, dysthymia or other depressive disorders not currently in the throes of a major depressive episode can be treated with DISTDP but require a more gradual access to their unconscious. One may or may not be able to access the core neurotic structure in a single interview. It may be necessary to have 2 or 3 interviews of a graded process. For patients with a low capacity to tolerate anxiety the emphasis is on bringing structural change to the discharge pattern of anxiety from the autonomic system to the striated muscle system. This is accomplished by systematically raising and lowering anxiety; and by fluidly moving between focus on current life and on the transference, following the lead of the patient's unconscious communications. In this way, capacity to tolerate anxiety is gradually increased as evidenced by increasing channeling of anxiety into the striated muscle system. Concomitantly, capacity to tolerate feelings is increased and communications become more meaningful. For depressed patients, the connection between feeling, anxiety and defense is not in operation. Feeling is instantly repressed into depressive symptoms and collapse. What is required here is bringing change in the defensive structure from instant repression of feeling into depressive symptoms to more obsessional defenses and to a striated muscle tension discharge pattern of anxiety, again with a graded technique. (Davanloo, 1990c,d,g,h; Whittemore, 1996). Following this brief, graded preparatory phase, these patients can enter into a course of DISTDP.

The majority of patients on the Spectrum of Psychoneurotic Disorders, who are highly resistant but have access to striated muscle discharge of anxiety, an intact defensive system and fusion of murderous rage and guilt occurring at age 4 or later, are candidates for the standard technique of DISTDP of 16-40 weekly sessions of an hour to an hour and a half duration (Davanloo, 1984, p.1466, 2005, p.2650, 2011). Patients with fusion at age 3 or earlier have complexities in their unconscious, which require a phase of Mobilization of the Unconscious, Multidimensional Unconscious Structural Changes and Psychoanalytic Investigation prior to commencing standard DISTDP. This can be a relatively straightforward process or a quite complex and lengthy one, depending on the specifics of the case. (Davanloo, 2010, 2011). Additional complications arise with the presence of one variety or another of unresolved Transference Neurosis from previous psychotherapies; in relational to other important figures in one's early family constellation (especially including intergenerational issues); or from relationships in one's professional life (Davanloo, 2009, 2010, 2011, 2012, 2013, 2014). Transference Neurosis in its various forms has been a major focus of Davanloo's training program and a detailed discussion will appear in the next chapter of this book.

Evidence Base for Davanloo's Metapsychology and ISTDP

Since 1975 Davanloo has presented his audio-visually recorded sessions with patients at annual conferences and courses. He has a large library of cases and case series representing the entire Spectrum of Psychoneurotic Disorders and of Fragility. Most of these cases also have outcome evaluation data. He reports in one case series, that of 617 consecutive general psychiatric patients presenting to the outpatient department at Montreal General Hospital, 28 percent were candidates for DISTDP. Of those 172 patients, 143 had successful outcomes. In a second series, with refinement of the technique to include patients with panic, somatization and functional disorders, the proportion suitable for DISTDP rose to 35 percent. Once he developed the technique to address fragility in the character, the proportion of patients suitable for DISTD rose to 52 percent (Davanloo, 2005, p. 2650).

Others have conducted and published over 25 outcome studies of ISTDP in one form or another. In many reviews and meta-analyses, studies of ISTDP were mixed with studies involving other short-term dynamic psychotherapies. A Cochrane review of ISTDP (Abbas et al, 2006), a meta-analysis of 21 outcome studies (Abbas et al, 2012), and reviews and meta-analyses for short-term dynamic psychotherapies (including ISTDP) for personality disorders (Town, 2011), depression (Driessen, 2010) and somatic disorders (Abbas, 2009) all conclude that ISTDP appears to be an effective treatment for this broad spectrum of patients.

CONCLUSION

I have attempted to provide a historical perspective and overview of Davanloo's pioneering work in short-term dynamic psychotherapy. The development of Davanloo's metapsychology was summarized. The spectrum of patients treatable with Davanloo's techniques was reviewed. The unconscious engine of psychoneurosis in Davanloo's metapsychology, namely the Psychopathological Dynamic Forces was highlighted. The role of unconscious Guilt and of Fusion in the Unconscious, the major destructive dynamic system at the nuclear structure of neurosis was discussed. In Davanloo's view, it is this destructive Fusion that is the source of masochism in the character and forms the major resistance to be reckoned with in psychotherapy. Trained in the psychoanalytic model Davanloo's early work utilized interpretation, especially of the link between current life, the past and the transference – the so-called T-C-P link. However, Davanloo has gone far beyond this model, based on his empiric observations and findings. His unique observations of the Neurobiological Pathways of Unconscious Anxiety, Murderous Rage, Guilt, Grief and Memory were presented. His techniques of Mobilization of the Unconscious, Total Removal of the Resistance and his Central Dynamic Sequence were briefly presented. Via the use of his techniques, Davanloo has been able to elucidate the complexity of the Unconscious and at the same time show the applicability of his techniques to a wider group of patients and complex clinical situations. The setting and duration of the types of DISTDP for particular patients, including certain complexities and complicating factors, was summarized and a brief review of the evidence base was provided.

Acknowledgment

Each of these topics is quite complex. A more detailed discussion goes far beyond the scope of this introduction. My aim was to clarify and outline the work to be done in further elaborating these important concepts. It has been a privilege to be able to participate in so many of the rich training activities that Dr. Davanloo has provided my colleagues and me. I hope this paper acts as an impetus for us all to share with our professional colleagues Dr. Davanloo's generous teaching. I am tremendously grateful to Dr. Davanloo for the contribution he has made to my life, both professionally and personally. I have been most fortunate to have Dr. Davanloo as a mentor and colleague for these past 25 years.

The theoretical concepts presented in these chapters including the terminology such as Mobilization of the Unconscious, Transference Component of the Resistance, Complex Transference Feeling, Unconscious Therapeutic Alliance, Central Dynamic Sequence, Perpetrator of the Unconscious, Fusion of Primitive Murderous Rage with Guilt and Sexuality, Intergenerational Destructive Competitive Transference Neurosis, Uplifting the Transference Neurosis, Unlocking the Unconscious, and others, are not mine. They were developed by Dr. Davanloo over the more than five decades of his systematic clinical research. My aim has been to integrate these concepts for my colleagues and to solidify my own understanding of them in the process. The work of Multidimensional Unconscious Structural Change is ongoing.

References

Abbas, A., Hancock, J., Henderson, J. and Kisely, S. (2006). Short-term psychodynamic psychotherapies for common mental disorders. *Cochrane Database Systematic Reviews.* Oct.18; (4): DOI: 10.1002/14651858. CD004687.pub3.

Abbas, A. (2009) Short-term psychodynamic psychotherapy for somatic disorders: a systematic review and meta-analysis of clinical trials. *Psychotherapy and Psychosomatics, 78* (5): 265–74.

Abbas, A., Town, J. and Driessen, E. (2012) Intensive short-term dynamic psychotherapy: a systematic review and meta-analysis of outcome research. *Harvard Review of Psychiatry,* 20 (2), 97-108.

Beeber, A. (1999a). The perpetrator of the unconscious in Davanloo's new metapsychology. Part I: Review of classic psychoanalytic concepts. *International Journal of Intensive Short-Term Dynamic Psychotherapy,* 13, 151-157.

Beeber, A. (1999b). The perpetrator of the unconscious in Davanloo's new metapsychology. Part II: Comparison of the perpetrator to classic psychoanalytic concepts. *International Journal of Intensive Short-Term Dynamic Psychotherapy,* 13, 159-176.

Beeber, A. (1999c). The perpetrator of the unconscious in Davanloo's new metapsychology. Part III: Specifics of Davanloo's technique. *International Journal of Intensive Short-Term Dynamic Psychotherapy,* 13, 177-189.

Davanloo, H. (1975) Proceedings of the First International Symposium and Workshop on Short-Term Dynamic Psychotherapy, Montreal, Canada. March 19-22.

Davanloo, H. (19776) Proceedings of the Second International Symposium and Workshops on Short-Term Dynamic Psychotherapy, Montreal, Canada. March 29-April 3.

Davanloo, H. (1977) Proceedings of the Third International Symposium and Workshops on Short-Term Dynamic Psychotherapy, Century Plaza, Los Angeles, California. November 9-13.

Davanloo, H. (1978) *Basic principles and techniques in short-term dynamic psychotherapy.* New York, NY. Spectrum Publications.

Davanloo, H. (1979a). Proceedings of the Audiovisual Symposium on Basic Principles of the Technique of Short-Term Dynamic Psychotherapy of Patients Suffering from Obsessional and Phobic Neurosis, Sheraton Hotel, New York, New York, March.

Davanloo, H. (1979b). Techniques in short-term dynamic psychotherapy. *Psychiatric Clinics of North America,* 2 (1), 11-21.

Davanloo, H. (Ed.) (1980a). *Short-term dynamic psychotherapy.* New York: J. Aronson.

Davanloo, H. (1980b). A method of short-term dynamic psychotherapy. In H. Davanloo (Ed.) *Short-term dynamic psychotherapy* (pp.43-71). New York: J. Aronson.

Davanloo, H. (1980c). The technique of crisis evaluation and intervention. In *Short-term dynamic psychotherapy* (pp. 245-281). New York: J. Aronson.

Davanloo, H. (1984). Short-Term Dynamic Psychotherapy. In *Kaplan and Sadock's comprehensive textbook of psychiatry* (4th ed., pp. 1460-1467). Philadelphia, Pa. Lippincott Williams and Wilkins.

Davanloo, H. (1990a). Clinical manifestations of super-ego pathology, Part I. In *Unlocking the unconscious: Selected papers of Habib Davanloo, MD* (pp. 163-192). Chichester, England: Wiley. (Reprinted from *International Journal of Short-Term Psychotherapy,* 2 (4)(1987), 225-254).

Davanloo, H. (1990b). Clinical manifestations of super-ego pathology, Part II. The resistance of the superego and the liberation of the paralyzed ego. In *Unlocking the unconscious: Selected papers of Habib Davanloo, MD* (pp. 193-216). (Reprinted from *International Journal of Short-Term Psychotherapy,* 3(1), (1988) 1-24).

Davanloo, H. (1990c). Intensive short-term dynamic psychotherapy with highly resistant depressed patients: Part I Restructuring the ego's regressive defenses. In *Unlocking the unconscious: Selected papers of Habib Davanloo, MD* (pp.47-80) (Reprinted from *International Journal of Short-Term Psychotherapy,* 2 (1987), 99-132).

Davanloo, H. (1990d). Intensive short-term dynamic psychotherapy with highly resistant depressed patients: Part II The Royal road to the unconscious. In *Unlocking the unconscious: Selected papers of Habib Davanloo, MD* (pp. 81-100) (Reprinted from *International Journal of Short-Term Psychotherapy,* 2 (1987), 167-185).

Davanloo, H. (1990e). The technique of unlocking the unconscious, Part I. In *Unlocking the unconscious: Selected papers of Habib Davanloo, MD* (pp. 101-124) (Reprinted from *International Journal of Short-Term Psychotherapy,* 3 (2) (1988), 99-121).

Davanloo, H. (1990f). The technique of unlocking the unconscious, Part II. Partial unlocking of the unconscious. In *Unlocking the unconscious: Selected papers of Habib Davanloo, MD* (pp. 125-162) (Reprinted from *International Journal of Short-Term Psychotherapy,* 3 (2) (1988), 123-159).

Davanloo, H. (1990g). The technique of unlocking the unconscious in patients suffering from functional disorders. Part I Restructuring ego's defenses. In *Unlocking the unconscious: Selected papers of Habib Davanloo, MD* (pp. 283-306) (Reprinted from *International Journal of Short-Term Psychotherapy,* 4 (2) (1989), 93-116).

Davanloo, H. (1990h). The technique of unlocking the unconscious in patients suffering from functional disorders. Part II Direct view of the dynamic unconscious. In *Unlocking the unconscious: Selected papers of Habib Davanloo, MD* (pp. 307-338) (Reprinted from *International Journal of Short-Term Psychotherapy,* 4 (2) (1989), 117-148).

Davanloo, H. (1990i). Intensive short-term dynamic psychotherapy with highly resistant patients: I. Handling resistance. In *Unlocking the unconscious: Selected papers of Habib Davanloo, MD* (pp.1-28) (Reprinted from *International Journal of Short-Term Psychotherapy,* 1 (2) (1986), 107-133).

Davanloo, H. (1990j) Proceedings of the 8th Annual Audiovisual Summer Institute on the Process of Working Through Intensive Short-Term Dynamic Psychotherapy, Part I. Killington, Vermont. July 18-21.

Davanloo, H. (1991) Proceedings of the 9th Annual Audiovisual Summer Institute on the Process of Working Through in Intensive Short-Term Dynamic Psychotherapy, Part II. Killington, Vermont. July 21-24.

Davanloo, H. (1993a). Proceedings of the Eleventh Annual Audiovisual Summer Institute on Intensive Short-Term Dynamic Psychotherapy. Treatment of Fragile Character Structure. Killington, Vermont. July.

Davanloo, H. (1993b). Proceedings of the Eleventh Annual Audiovisual Immersion Course on Intensive Short-Term Dynamic Psychotherapy. Treatment of Fragile Character Structure. Bad Ragaz, Switzerland. December.

Davanloo, H. (1998). Proceedings of the Seventeenth Annual Audiovisual Exploration of the Unconscious. Technical and Metapsychological Roots of Davanloo's Psychoanalytic Technique. Technique and Metapsychology of the Process of Working Through: Fragile Character Structure. Montreal, Canada. November.

Davanloo, H. (2000a). Intensive short-term dynamic psychotherapy Spectrum of psychoneurotic disorders. *Intensive short-term dynamic psychotherapy: Selected papers of Habib Davanloo, MD*. (pp.1-36) Chichester, England: Wiley. (Reprinted from *International Journal of Short-Term Psychotherapy,* 10(3/4) (1995), 121-155).

Davanloo, H. (2000b). Intensive short-term dynamic psychotherapy Technique of partial and major unlocking of the unconscious with a highly resistant patient. Part I Partial unlocking In *Intensive short-term dynamic psychotherapy: Selected papers of Habib Davanloo, MD*. (pp.37-61) Chichester, England: Wiley. (Reprinted from *International Journal of Short-Term Psychotherapy,* 10(3/4) (1995), 157-181).

Davanloo, H. (2000c). Intensive short-term dynamic psychotherapy Technique of partial and major unlocking of the unconscious. Part II The course of the trial therapy after partial unlocking. In *Intensive short-term dynamic psychotherapy: Selected papers of Habib Davanloo, MD*. (pp.63-110) Chichester, England: Wiley. (Reprinted from *International Journal of Short-Term Psychotherapy,* 10(3/4) (1995), 183-230.

Davanloo, H. (2000d). Management of tactical defenses in intensive short-term dynamic psychotherapy. Part I. Overview, tactical defenses of cover words and indirect speech. In *Intensive short-term dynamic psychotherapy: Selected papers of Habib Davanloo, MD*. (pp.111-134) Chichester, England: Wiley. (Reprinted from *International Journal of Short-Term Psychotherapy,* 11(3) (1996), 129-152).

Davanloo, H. (2000e). Management of tactical defenses in intensive short-term dynamic psychotherapy. Part II. Spectrum of tactical defenses. In *Intensive short-term dynamic psychotherapy: Selected papers of Habib Davanloo, MD*. (pp.135-182) Chichester, England: Wiley. (Reprinted from *International Journal of Short-Term Psychotherapy,* 11(3), (1996) 153-199).

Davanloo, H. (2000f). Intensive short-term dynamic psychotherapy – central dynamic sequence: phase of pressure. In *Intensive short-term dynamic psychotherapy: Selected papers of Habib Davanloo, MD*. (pp.183-208) Chichester, England: Wiley. (Reprinted from *International Journal of Short-Term Psychotherapy,* 13 (4), (1999) 211-236).

Davanloo, H. (2000g). Intensive short-term dynamic psychotherapy – central dynamic sequence: phase of challenge. In *Intensive short-term dynamic psychotherapy: Selected papers of Habib Davanloo, MD*. (pp.209-234) Chichester, England: Wiley. (Reprinted from *International Journal of Short-Term Psychotherapy,* 13 (4), (1999) 237-262).

Davanloo, H. (2000h). Intensive short-term dynamic psychotherapy – central dynamic sequence: head on collision with resistance. In *Intensive short-term dynamic psychotherapy: Selected papers of Habib Davanloo, MD*. (pp.235-253) Chichester, England: Wiley. (Reprinted from *International Journal of Short-Term Psychotherapy,* 13 (4), (1999) 263-282).

Davanloo, H. (2000) *Intensive short-term dynamic psychotherapy: Selected papers of Habib Davanloo, MD*. Chichester, England: Wiley.

Davanloo, H. (2001) Intensive short-term dynamic psychotherapy: Extended major direct access to the unconscious. *European Psychotherapy,* 2 (2) 25-70.

single session using the standard format of Davanloo's Intensive Short-Term Dynamic Psychotherapy (DISTDP) in those with early Fusion. What is necessary is a preliminary, more extensive process of Mobilization of the Unconscious and a focus on Multidimensional Unconscious Structural Change (MDUSC) before one can access the Original Neurosis directly and begin a traditional course of DISTDP (Davanloo, 2013, 2014). A further complexity arises with the presence of one or another form of Transference Neurosis in the Unconscious of the patient. Many psychotherapists are familiar with notion of a persistent, unresolved Transference Neurosis as a complication of previous therapies. However Davanloo has identified other important sources of Transference Neurosis which, when present, serve as a major obstacle to the breakdown of Fusion in the Unconscious. The presence of Transference Neurosis serves as a morbid defensive system that renders the Original Neurosis inaccessible. The identification, understanding and management of Transference Neurosis in DISTDP will be the major focus of this chapter.

Classic Psychoanalytic View

Transference

The foundation of any psychoanalytically oriented psychotherapy rests on the principles of Transference and Resistance. Transference can be defined as the phenomena of experiencing feelings, drives or fantasies towards a person in the present which are inappropriate to that person, and really apply to another person, usually from the person's past (Greenson, 1967). It often involves the repetition or displacement of reactions that originate with significant figures in early childhood (Freud, 1905, 1912, 1916-17). Though first observed by Freud in the psychoanalytic relationship, Transference can occur in any interpersonal relationship in current life. It often involves both "positive" and "negative" valence. When present in psychoanalysis and psychotherapy, Transference can be a vehicle for therapy or can function as a resistance to remembering (and experiencing) the past. Therapists must be prepared to be exposed to the powerful positive and negative feelings engendered in Transference phenomena (Chessick, 2002).

Countertransference

Therapists are not immune to experiencing Transference reactions. When Transference phenomena occur in the therapist during psychotherapy it is called Countertransference. Countertransference may be as a result of some specific issue in the patient that activates a reaction in therapist's unconscious (Racker, 1968). However, it may also result primarily from a specific unresolved conflict in the Unconscious of the therapist. Mostly, it is viewed as a phenomena contributed to jointly by the patient and therapist. When the therapist is aware of their Countertransference, it can be a useful tool for understanding the patient's Unconscious (Gabbard, 1999).

Transference Neurosis

It was Freud's view, that when the Transference was handled properly, Transference Neurosis developed. He viewed Transference Neurosis as "a new edition of the old disease" (Freud, 1916-17). The Original Neurosis, along with later variations, is "replaced" by a new neurosis in the Transference. It is characterized by intense transference feelings such that the analyst becomes the central focus of the patient's life. The analyst becomes an extremely important object relationship determined by projections of split off self and object representations (Chessick, 2007). In classical psychoanalysis, it has been the view that the Transference Neurosis, and thereby, the Original Neurosis, could be "cured" by working through via the process of (transference) interpretation (Greenson, 1965). The infantile neurosis is revived in the Transference but not in a one to one manner. It is influenced by events and relationships over the years before the analysis so as to involve what Chessick called a "layering" quality. It often has a shifting, dynamic quality, involves regression and repetition, and becomes a resistance itself in analysis. It is the working through of the Transference Neurosis by interpretation that differentiates classic psychoanalysis form other forms of treatment (Chessick, 2002, p. 88).

The classic analysts restricted their interventions to questions and interpretations. Anything else was considered a "parameter" (Eissler, 1953). The strict adherence to this role, viewed by many as a caricature of Freud's technique, served to maximize the formation of Transference Neurosis but had its limitations and complications. As Psychoanalysis evolved over the years, other therapeutic factors were emphasized including the "Corrective

Emotional Experience (Alexander, 1980)," the "Therapeutic Alliance" (Zetzel 1956), and the "Working Alliance" (Greenson, 1965). Though analytic candidates were initially required to have cases of Transference Neurosis for the certification of their training, many were said to have had difficulty finding such cases. It was felt, too, that analytic patients with primarily characterologic problems often didn't develop Transference Neurosis. Chessick noted that frequently, even in formal psychoanalysis Transference Neurosis did not appear. Furthermore, when it did appear, it was "not always a reason to be jubilant." He felt that patients with impaired defensive structures were not able to utilize the interpretation of Transference Neurosis to work through intrapsychic difficulties. Some Transference Neuroses did not respond to interpretation at all and bordered on "Transference Psychosis" (Chessick, 2002 pp. 87-89). Failure of the Transference Neurosis to resolve via interpretation, either because of the dynamics of the patient or as Davanloo maintains, from the lack of effectiveness of interpretation per se, can result in a persistent iatrogenic Transference Neurosis, therapeutic stalemate and interminable treatment. There developed a building consensus among analysts that Transference Neurosis was not necessary for successful analysis or training. Often difficult to identify, it became viewed more like a quantitatively intense Transference reaction. Brenner called Transference Neurosis a "tautology, the concept is an anachronism." He felt that a transference manifestation was dynamically indistinguishable from a transference neurotic symptom and that to call it Transference Neurosis was to add a "word without meaning. Transference is enough. Nothing is gained by expanding the term to transference neurosis." He called for abandonment of the term (Brenner, 1982). Cooper shared this view and called Transference Neurosis a "Concept Ready for Retirement" (Cooper, 1987).

CONTRIBUTIONS OF HABIB DAVANLOO

Historical Background

For a more detailed review of the development of Davanloo's metapsychology and methods of psychotherapy see the preceding chapter (Beeber, 2016). Freud initially viewed the development of Transference Neurosis desirable in a successful psychoanalysis. However, he became concerned with the increasing length of psychoanalysis. Freud felt that the "unconscious sense of guilt" representing the "superego's resistance" was the "most powerful factor, and the one most dreaded by us" (Freud, 1926). He identified patients in whom there was a "force defending itself by every possible means against recovery and which is absolutely resolved to hold on to illness and suffering." He attributed a portion of this force to the unconscious need for suffering and punishment emanating from what he termed the punitive superego. However he came to believe when looking at this "negative therapeutic reaction" and at masochism in the character, that, in contrast to the pleasure principle, there must also be at work in the unconscious, a destructive instinct "which we trace back to the original death instinct of living matter." It was upon taking this view that Freud concluded, "For the moment we must bow to the superiority of the forces against which we see out efforts come to nothing. Even to exert a psychical influence on simple masochism is a severe tax upon our powers" (Freud, 1937). Davanloo noted Freud's concerns but concluded that Freudian psychoanalysis bypassed the resistances of the superego, further lengthening the course of psychoanalysis. Some cases became interminable with persistent unresolved Transference Neurosis.

Trained in the classic psychoanalytic tradition, Davanloo became troubled by this ever-increasing length of psychoanalysis. He presented his initial attempts at shortening the course of therapy most prominently in his first three international symposia on short-term dynamic psychotherapy (Davanloo, 1975, 1976, 1977). He characterized his technique as emphasizing the importance of the therapeutic alliance generated by a dynamic interaction between the patient and the therapist. His technique employed active utilization of the transference relationship, with active interpretation of transference resistance and the active avoidance of a transference neurosis. He observed, based on more than a hundred early cases, that core neurosis could be de-repressed and experienced deeply in the first few sessions. Further, by bringing insight into the relationship between impulse-feeling/anxiety/defense and transference/current life/past one could achieve rapid and permanent changes in symptom disturbances and characterological difficulties (Davanloo, 1980).

While Freud bypassed the resistances of the "hostile superego," others in the field of short-term dynamic psychotherapy avoided superego resistance by the application of selection criteria that excluded such patients. Patients were typically selected for having a circumscribed focus to their difficulties, high motivation, positive response to interpretation and absence of superego resistance (Sifneos, 1980, Marmor, 1980, Malan, 1980). In contrast, Davanloo sought to increase the range of patients suitable for short-term dynamic psychotherapy.

The majority of patients seen in his clinic and practice were more complex than those patients typically selected by his colleagues for short-term therapies. They often had multifocal symptom disturbances, complexity in their character structure often of a syntonic nature, and masochistic self-defeating character traits. Davanloo noted that this group of patients evidenced resistances of the "superego." He elaborated the dynamics of superego pathology in great detail using audio-visually recorded sessions from a series of cases (Davanloo, 1990a,b) He later developed the concept of "Perpetrator of the Unconscious" to describe this destructive dynamic system (Davanloo, 2000a,b). A review traces Davanloo's development of this concept and his technique to address it (Beeber, 1999a,b,c).

Undaunted by Freud's pessimism, he sought to develop an approach that didn't rely on "slow demolition" via interpretation. Through the extensive use of audiovisual recording of his sessions with this wider range of patients he painstakingly developed his techniques of "the Central Dynamic Sequence," (Davanloo, 2001, 2005) "Mobilization of the Unconscious" (Davanloo, 2007-2015), "De-Fusion of Primitive Murderous Rage, Guilt and Sexuality" (Davanloo, 2009), and "Total Removal of Resistance" (Davanloo, 2007-2015, 2010-2014). With total removal of resistance and the mobilization of the triple factors of the Transference Component of the Resistance, the Complex Transference Feelings, and the Unconscious Therapeutic Alliance, direct experience of all of the mixed feelings in relation to the key psychogenetic figure(s) become accessible in a single session. This provides a direct view of the psychopathological dynamic forces in the unconscious, which can now be integrated by the patient. From there, the processes of "Psychoanalytic Investigation" and "Multidimensional Unconscious Structural Change" proceed (Davanloo, 2010, 2011, 2012 2013, 2014). By virtue of the development of his techniques, Davanloo has been able to successfully apply his method to the very group of patients that have been bypassed by both psychoanalysis and other short-term techniques.

Davanloo's Expanded View of Transference Neurosis

All of these observations are Davanloo's, not mine. I have had the privilege to be supervised and trained by Davanloo beginning in 1991 and continuing to the present. Most of what I present below comes from unpublished work of Davanloo's, generously shared with us in his Training Workshops (Davanloo, 2007-2015) and International Symposia (Davanloo,

2007-2015) where I have had the honor of being invited to present from 2007 to 2015. I am deeply indebted to him for his generous sharing of his unique observations and his synthesis of the metapsychology of the unconscious and for giving me permission to use material from the workshops and symposia in this publication. Davanloo's clinical research concerning Transference Neurosis began in 1976 and continues to the present. He has observed many cases of patients who suffer from a Transference Neurosis in relationship to a previous therapist, many of which have been presented in his supervisory training programs [I refer here only to those programs to which I had the privilege of attending (Davanloo, 1991-1993, 1997-2005) but other training programs share the same experience]. The presence of a persistent Transference Neurosis that has not been sufficiently worked through, leads to an impairment of the patient's original defensive structure. Providing an additional morbid defensive system, the Transference Neurosis renders the original normal defenses non functional and renders the Original Neurosis and Fusion of Murderous Rage/Guilt/Sexuality inaccessible. The Original Fusion and the effect of Transference Neurosis are represented schematically in Figures 1 and 2.

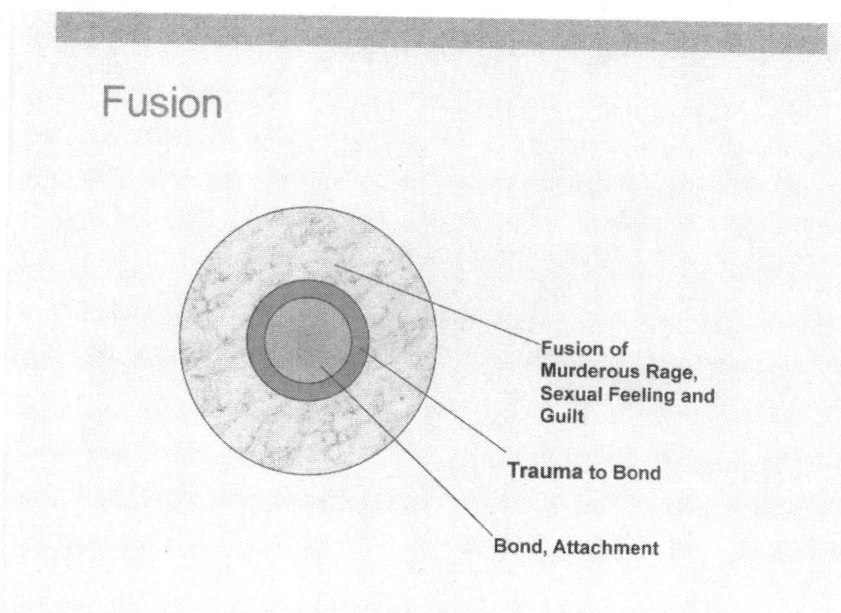

Adapted from Davanloo, 2009. Used with permission of the author.

Figure 1. Fusion of Primitive Murderous Rage and Guilt.

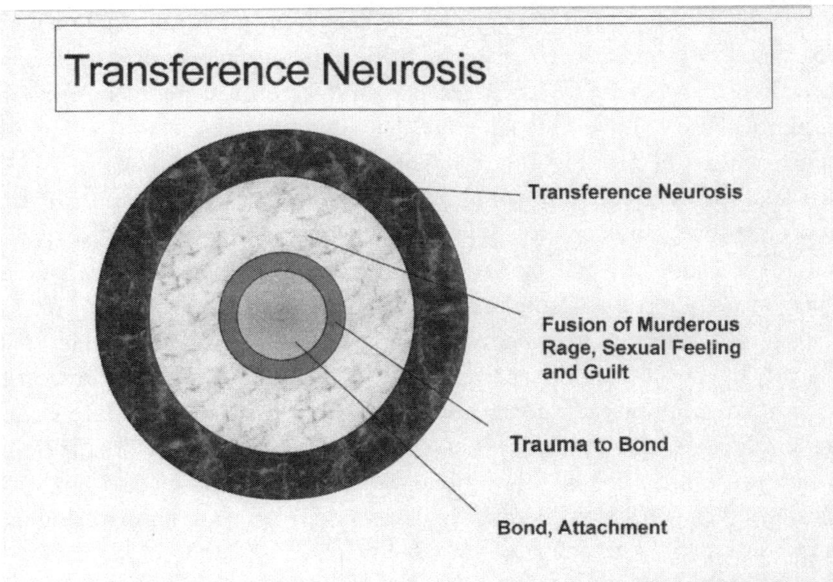

Adapted from Davanloo, 2007-2015. Used with permission of the author.

Figure 2. Transference Neurosis.

These are cases of what might be considered formal Transference Neurosis - that is Transference Neurosis developed in the course of therapy. However, Davanloo has offered a unique conceptualization of Transference Neurosis that goes far beyond the idea of the formal Transference Neurosis. He noted that Transference Neurosis was not limited to the patient therapist relationship. Just as Transference and Counter Transference can occur in any relationship, so too can Transference Neurosis, should the quality and quantity of the mutual Transference reactions achieve the necessary intensity. This will be elaborated further.

In the mid-1990's Davanloo introduced a format of therapy called "Major Extended Mobilization of the Unconscious." He used this powerful technique for professionals who were in training in his techniques, in a the form of a block of three full days duration set 1-3 months apart (Davanloo, 2005). He also has, over the years, conducted a number of training workshops for groups of professionals studying his techniques. One such group, instituted in 2007, is the Montreal Closed-Circuit Experiential Training Workshops in the Mobilization of the Unconscious and DISTDP. This program continues to the present (Davanloo, 2007-2016). I am most fortunate to have had the privilege of participating in this program from 2007 through 2014. The purpose of the experiential training is the learning of the technique of Mobilization of the Unconscious. The main focus is the identification of unconscious resistances in the trainee. The group typically consists of 8-12 professionals, meeting six to eight hours a day for four to six days. The program consists of a mixture of didactic review of metapsychology with heavy emphasis on the use of audiovisual-recorded material from Davanloo's teaching and research library and of interviews from previous workshops. Members of the workshop also conduct live Closed Circuit observed and recorded interviews of each other, one person in the "patient" role and the other in the "therapist" role. Through this process of the use live, observed and recorded sessions, of interviews conducted by Dr. Davanloo as well, and of extensive review of recorded material it has been possible for members of the program to come face to face with the role resistance in their own unconscious plays in their work. They are then in a position to begin to bring changes in their unconscious in multiple dimensions. What became obvious in the workshops was that Transference Neurosis was playing a major role in complicating the unconscious defensive system of many of the participants. This led to an emphasis being placed on Transference Neurosis. Presentations from this program have been delivered at Davanloo's symposia in Montreal from 2007 to the present. Transference Neurosis is currently a central focus of these annual Audio-Visual Symposia on the Mobilization of the Unconscious (Davanloo, 2000-2015).

What Davanloo noted, in his clinical work and in his training workshops, was that the phenomena of transferring a neurosis from one person to another was not unique to the psychoanalytic relationship. Transference is a two way street in any close relationship. If one then takes the view that Transference Neurosis as a *transferred neurosis*, i.e., a neurosis transferred from one person's unconscious to another's, one sees the same process in many different relationships. He noted that when transference phenomena were qualitatively and quantitatively sufficient, they had the same impact on the defensive structure of the patient, as would a formal Transference Neurosis in the therapeutic setting. He has presented numerous audio-video recorded sessions with patients and with members of the training workshops demonstrating the many variations that Transference Neurosis could take. For example, one may see transference phenomena with a spouse or with a child. In this situation, the husband relates to his wife as if she is his mother, or the wife relates to the husband as if he is her father or mother, for that matter. When the transfer of neurosis involves one's children, the parent relates to the child as if they were their own parent (or grandparent). As with the unresolved formal Transference Neurosis, Fusion of murderous rage/guilt/sexual feeling originating in one person's unconscious can be transferred to the unconscious of the other person, resulting in a new Fusion and new neurosis on top of the Original Neurosis. The defensive system becomes impaired and direct access to the Original Neurosis and Fusion is not possible.

The Closed-Circuit workshop, given its intensity, is a laboratory for the study of these phenomena. With the use of audio-visually recorded and observed interviews in the training workshops Davanloo has elucidated the most common types of Transference Neurosis. Each type will be taken in turn (Davanloo, 2007-2016, 2007-2015).

1. Unresolved Transference Neurosis from Prior Therapy

In a DISTDP practice one often encounters patients who have had prior therapy, (either ISTDP or therapy of another type). In many cases the patient has formed an intense transference to the previous therapist, which was insufficiently worked through. This Transference Neurosis is often of a dependent nature. Even if the prior therapy was ISTDP, which strives to avoid Transference Neurosis, major technical errors on the part of the therapist may have prevented sufficient rise in the Transference Component of the Resistance and the Complex Transference Feelings to protect the process from development of Transference Neurosis. Unconscious issues in the previous therapist often play an important role. Conflicted relationships with one or both parents, with grandparents or with siblings may unconsciously contribute to the therapist manipulating the transference by introducing issues from their own unconscious. This is especially prominent if Fusion in the therapist's unconscious occurs in very early life (age 3 or younger). In its most exaggerated form, the therapist bulldozes the patient by telling the patient what to focus on rather than following the lead of the Unconscious Therapeutic Alliance. The therapist may have access to malignant defenses, defending against their own unconscious guilt by acting out. In its worst form the therapist may actually have psychopathic traits. In this situation the process may resemble brainwashing. The presence of a history of multiple therapists may compound all of these issues (Davanloo, 2007-2016, 2007-2015).

2. Result of Professional Work

In Davanloo's training workshops, the aim is to identify and work through unconscious resistances that impede one's psychotherapeutic work. A common defensive structure encountered is the presence of Transference Neurosis as a result of one's professional work, such as an extremely busy practice with highly complex patients. Oftentimes, the workshop member may have a DISTDP practice of up to 10 hours a week while also being in full time employment with difficult patients, such as in a forensic setting with psychopathic patients; or in a clinic or hospital setting with borderline patients and patients suffering from psychotic disorders. With insufficient time for reflection, rest or relaxation, there is little opportunity to process ones own unconscious reactions. Issues in the patients' unconscious are transferred to or activate certain issues in the therapist's unconscious. In each instance, a seemingly minor problem festers and in a year's time becomes a major issue in the unconscious of the therapist (Davanloo, 2007-2016, 2007-2015).

3. Occurring in Professional Relationships

Another form of Transference Neurosis seen in the training workshops is a Transference Neurosis that occurs in professional relationships. A colleague or coworker becomes a transference figure. Issues in the unconscious of the workshop member are projected and transferred to the colleague or vice versa. The colleague now assumes a position that is psychologically larger than life. This person may be idealized, or devalued and despised. With respect to a primary supervisor, or training director the situation commonly seen is one of identification and idealization. If the supervisor themself has certain unconscious issues in relation to their own family, or has psychopathic traits, these issues can be projected onto the trainee. In the context of the trainee identifying with and idealizing the supervisor, a Transference Neurosis can ensue. What happens in this situation is that a new Fused Neurosis occurs on top of the Original Fusion (Davanloo, 2007-2016, 2007-2015).

4. Intergenerational Transference Neurosis

The Intergenerational Transmission of Transference Neurosis is the most common form of Transference Neurosis seen in the training workshops (Davanloo, 2007-2016). As mentioned repeatedly, Neurosis, which in Davanloo's metapsychology is a result of Fusion of Murderous Rage, Guilt and Sexuality in the Unconscious, can be transferred from one person to another in any close relationship. Transfer to family members is extremely common. It is often seen in marital relationships with one partner or the other projecting issues from their unconscious originating with a parent and transferring the neurotic constellation to the spouse. This process can span generations as well. Intergenerational Transference Neurosis often begins in the earliest days of life, with Fusion taking place typically by age 3 or earlier. The infant is a sponge for the incorporation, introjection and identification of feelings originating with parents and grandparents. The young, undeveloped defensive system is characterized by projection, projective identification and idealization. Projective anxiety is heavy. In this context, the infant can't distinguish its own feelings from those of the other. Anxiety is at the level of fear of destroying the other or of being destroyed. The parent or grandparent can easily transfer his or her own neurosis to the infant. A common dynamic in operation in this setting involves destructive competiveness in one generation being transferred to another generation. A typical example involves a parent, having issues of competition with one of their parents or siblings for the love and affection of the other parent. This competiveness takes on a destructive dimension (murderous rage fused with guilt), not just to best the other but also to destroy the other. This destructive competitiveness can then transferred to one's spouse. The spouse is then related to as if they are a figure from the past. Then the infant or child is brought into the arena and becomes the repository for the destructive competitiveness. From early life the child is turned against one parent by the other. An example of his complex situation involves a mother who has been turned against her siblings by her father or mother. She marries and ultimately transfers this destructive competitiveness to her spouse. She then turns her son against his father as a transfer of the neurosis originating in the previous generation. This can be compounded further if the marital relationship ends in divorce, death or even suicide. The child via this intergenerational transfer of neurosis has been turned against an innocent person, his father. This then leads to the development of an extremely high degree of unconscious guilt, which in turn fuels further destructiveness (often self-destructiveness) and masochism in the character (Davanloo, 2007-2016, 2007-2015).

5. *Combined Intergenerational Transference Neurosis Plus Transference Neurosis from Previous Therapy*

It is not uncommon to see a combined form of Transference Neurosis. The person who is the repository of Intergenerational Transference Neurosis experiences an especially heavy load of unconscious guilt. This leads to the need to perpetuate ones suffering through maintaining the Transference Neurosis. With ever increasing self-destructiveness, there is further susceptibility to and searching for additional new Transference Neuroses. If one enters into therapy there is an exceedingly strong need to sabotage the therapy and develop another Transference Neurosis. Now there are two new Fusions on top of the Original Fusion (Davanloo, 2007-2016, 2007-2015).

SUSCEPTIBILITY TO TRANSFERENCE NEUROSIS

In his audio-visual recorded case series research Davanloo has identified several factors that contribute to one's susceptibility to develop Transference Neurosis. This applies equally to the clinical situation and to the professional setting. The presence of early and extensive trauma to the affectionate bond to parents is an important and frequent risk factor. When fusion occurs before the age of four, especially at age one or two, the defensive system is not yet fully developed. Defenses consist mainly of projection, introjection and projective identification. Obsessional defenses are not yet well formed. When this early Fusion is coupled with Intergenerational Transmission of Neurosis from a parent or grandparent, the young child is under the impact of extremely heavy unconscious guilt. Further susceptibility arises if one or more of the figures in early life have tendencies to act out or have psychopathic traits. The masochistic need to suffer and be punished becomes very high. The need to repetitively sabotage and punish the self becomes deeply entrenched in the character and manifests itself into adulthood. Often when such a person attempts to obtain help or psychotherapy they do so in a self-sabotaging and self-damaging way. It is not uncommon for them to gravitate to therapists who themselves suffer from early Fusion and Intergenerational Transference Neurosis and who may even have psychopathic traits. Early Fusion in the patient coupled with early Fusion in the therapist (projected onto the patient) is a recipe for Transference Neurosis (Davanloo, 2007-2016, 2007-2015).

INDICATIONS OF THE PRESENCE OF TRANSFERENCE NEUROSIS

In the psychotherapeutic setting, one notes that "normal," expected character defenses are not operating. Obsessional defenses are absent and are replaced by a set of malignant character defenses, most often projection, projective identification and compliance/defiance. One frequently sees the presence of oppositional and psychopathic character traits. With this impairment in the defensive organization, "normal" defenses are not working and there is an associated high level of unconscious anxiety, mainly in the form of projective anxiety. This is accompanied by a relatively lower capacity to tolerate anxiety manifested by the person being flooded with anxiety in certain interpersonal situations, most notably in the Transference relationship.

In the DISTDP setting, when one attempts the process of "Mobilization" or "Total Removal of the Resistance" one rapidly notices that efforts to mobilize the Transference Component of the Resistance fall into difficulty in the presence of Transference Neurosis. This occurs despite otherwise adequate technical knowledge and skill. At this point the therapist should become suspicious of the presence of Transference Neurosis.

This issue is especially prominent in the Closed-Circuit Audio-Visual observation and supervision in Davanloo's training workshops. The inability to obtain the expected mobilization of Transference Component of the Resistance can implicate a Transference Neurosis in either the interviewee or the interviewer. In this setting, when the interviewer, in the "therapist" role, has a Transference Neurosis, they often have great difficulty applying Davanloo's most powerful intervention, the Head-On-Collision with the Destructive Organization of the Resistance. Despite specific supervision to apply the Head on Collision and despite adequate knowledge and skill the interviewer either bypasses the Head-On-Collision completely, or applies it in such a way as to water down or undo its effectiveness, thereby avoiding mobilizing their own unconscious. Difficulty applying the Head-On-Collision is a strong indicator of Transference Neurosis on the part of the interviewer (Davanloo, 2007-2016, 2007-2015).

EFFECTS OF TRANSFERENCE NEUROSIS ON THE CHARACTER

All of the forms of Transference Neurosis enumerated above have profound effects on the character structure. As mentioned, the presence of Transference Neurosis leads to an extremely high degree of unconscious guilt, which in turns fuels destructiveness and masochism in the character. This can rise to the level of "moral masochism" manifested by an addiction, so to speak, to perpetual suffering. The normal defensive system is impaired and gives way to malignant character defenses. These defenses are inadequate in daily life and the person becomes flooded with anxiety, often of a projective quality. They become symptomatic with anxiety often with an autonomic discharge pattern. Lastly, there is significant impairment of memory, most importantly affecting memory involving close relationships with figures in the past (Davanloo, 2007-2016, 2007-2015). For professionals, the presence of one form or another of Transference Neurosis in their unconscious has serious consequences. It can be a major obstacle in their work. What is more, they are susceptible to passing on the Transference Neurosis to those they set out to help.

Davanloo's Technique of Total Removal of Transference Neurosis

The standard format of DISTDP involves the utilization of Davanloo's Central Dynamic Sequence. For a detailed discussion see the previous chapter (Beeber, 2016). Briefly, the application of pressure leads to tilting characterologic defenses in the dimension of the transference. With the addition first of passing challenge, and then systematic challenge added to the pressure, resistance becomes crystallized in the transference, which leads to mobilization of the Transference Component of the Resistance. Head-on-collision with the Transference Resistance sets the stage for the actual experience of the Complex Transference Feeling, the triggering mechanism that de-fuses unconscious murderous rage from unconscious guilt (and sexual feelings). The Unconscious Therapeutic Alliance is concomitantly mobilized and all the mixed feelings in relation to the psychogenetic figure are experienced. There then is a direct view of the core neurotic structure, the Original Neurosis. The presence of Transference Neurosis, in one form or another, either alone or in combination, serves as a new Fusion on top of the Original Fusion. It becomes very difficult, if not impossible, to get sufficient mobilization of the Transference Component of the Resistance to break down the Fusion. It is critical to be able to recognize the presence of Transference Neurosis in this situation. Once the presence of Transference Neurosis is established, a modification of the Central Dynamic Sequence is necessary. The process shifts to inquiry into the relationship with the Transference Neurosis figure (e.g., professional colleague, previous therapist, training supervisor). As the exploration continues feelings in relationship to that person are mobilized. This in turn mobilizes anxiety and defense. Pressure to the avoided feelings towards that person is applied, often coupled with Head-On-Collision which leads to the beginning of the mobilization of the Neurobiological Pathway of Murderous Rage. When the person begins to show signs of experiencing the rage, one then shifts the process to the Transference. This is a crucial intervention and the optimum timing is critical. Davanloo has shown in many cases that if one keeps the focus here with the Transference Neurosis figure, that even with heavy experience of the Murderous Rage, with activation of the Neurobiological pathway, the transfer of visual imagery to the genetic figure often does not take place, and guilt is then not experienced. The person may feel that the rage is "justified," no connection to the Original Neurosis is obtained and the Original Fusion remains. However, if at that critical moment of activation of the Neurobiological Pathway of Murderous Rage the therapist or interviewer shifts the process, the focus on the Transference serves to mobilize the Unconscious further. At this point, one says something along the lines of: "This may be difficult for you to do but if you take all those feelings towards "X" and you direct them at me, in your thoughts and ideas- not actually do it; but in your ideas, how would you unleash those feelings at me? … How viciously? If you totally unleashed further…" Typically what ensues is the temporary break down of Fusion. The actual experience of the Neurobiological Pathway of the Primitive Murderous Rage is heavily experienced in the here and now. The person sees a vivid image of the dead body of the therapist/interviewer. The damage is seen in full detail. With focus on the eyes of the murdered therapist/interviewer the visual image is transferred to the visual image of a figure from the person's early life- someone who is dynamically linked to the Transference Neurosis. Intense Guilt-laden Unconscious feelings are mobilized and experienced. This passage of the Guilt-laden feelings may last for from five to ten minutes or more, followed by the experience of positive and Grief-laden feelings in relation to the psychogenetic figure. This then affords a direct connection of the early figure to the Transference Neurosis figure. A phase of repetitive analysis of the process further consolidates the connection to the Transference Neurosis. A formal Transference Neurosis can be worked through sufficiently to allow access to the Original Fusion, in a series of several (2-6) sessions.

However the presence of the Intergenerational Destructive Competitive Transference Neurosis is another matter. Davanloo reports that the analysis of his data from the training workshops indicates that with those who have an Intergenerational Destructive Competitive form of Transference Neurosis, after the Breakthrough into the Unconscious, and De-fusion, there is a return of the resistance in the next session (Davanloo, 2015). The presence of the Intergenerational Transference Neurosis has impaired the person's defensive system. Restructuring of the defensive system from malignant character defenses to a "normal" defensive system is necessary. Projective anxiety is high. The Neurobiological Pathway of Primitive Murderous Rage is not fully accessed. As a result the pathway of the connection via the eyes from the Transference to the genetic figure does not operate sufficiently, visual imagery is impaired, memory is impaired, and the experience of guilt is not of sufficient intensity to permanently remove the Transference Neurosis.

What is needed in these situations is the systematic application on the process of Multidimensional Unconscious Structural Change (Davanloo, 2012, 2013). Immediately after the breakthrough has taken place, systematic analysis of the projective anxiety, the malignant defenses, and their effect on the experience of the Neurobiological Pathways needs to take place. As the capacity to tolerate anxiety is increased, and projective anxiety is diminished and ultimately eliminated, malignant character defenses give way to more obsessional defenses. Memory, often of a multisensory type (visual imagery, smells, tastes and sensations from the past) dramatically improves. Working through requires repetitive breakthroughs. The therapists/interviewers need to be fluid in their technique, shifting focus in synchrony with the Unconscious Therapeutic Alliance. This is a difficult art to master and is impeded by the presence of Fusion in the therapist's/interviewer's unconscious. The therapist needs to be skilled in the utilization of what Davanloo calls the projective technique. This involves selecting a focus based on signals from the Unconscious Therapeutic Alliance, which is highly conflictual for the person, is avoided and heavily mobilizes the Transference Component of the Resistance. One might pick up on an issue from a previous session and utilize it to apply pressure to the avoided feeling by the use of fantasy. This can apply to aggressive feelings, positive feelings or feelings of a sexual nature. Pressure to the avoided feeling, coupled with Head-On-Collision, mobilizes unconscious resistance further. The avoided feeling, Transference Component of the Resistance, and the Complex Transference Feeling are now well mobilized. In a sense, the process is similar to that used to mobilize feeling towards the Transference Neurosis figure. For further discussion of Davanloo's method of treatment for Transference Neurosis see the recent publications of Hickey (2015,2015a).

With repeated breakthroughs, the intensity of the actual experience of the Neurobiological Pathway of the Primitive Murderous Rage increases until it is experienced at an optimum level. This is associated with a concomitant increase in the intensity of the experience of Guilt-laden feelings, which hastens the draining of the Pathogenic Reservoir of Unconscious Guilt. Throughout the process an emphasis is placed on the role that guilt plays in perpetuating suffering through maintaining the Transference Neurosis. Guilt is especially heavy in the Intergenerational Transference Neurosis because what is often the case is that an "innocent," loved person has become the target of one's murderous rage. This high level of guilt fuels the self-destructiveness and addiction to suffering and leads to susceptibility to or even seeking out further Transference Neuroses. If left untouched, the destructive organization of the resistance fueled by and fueling the Transference Neurosis, in a vicious cycle, maintains an impaired defensive system and can even lead to psychopathic traits. However, when the process of Multidimensional Unconscious Structural Change has been successful (often requiring a dozen or more sessions), access to the Original Neurosis via the standard technique of DISTDP is now possible (Davanloo, 2007-2016, 2007-2015).

CONCLUSION

Davanloo was a pioneer in developing several techniques to shorten the course of psychoanalytic therapies. He also developed a powerful teaching and learning format in the form of Closed-Circuit Audio-visual training. He adapted the closed-circuit training to a structure in the form of experiential workshops designed to address unconscious resistance on the part of the therapist – resistances that served as obstacles to one's work. This interest intersected with his interest in preventing and eliminating Transference Neurosis. In his clinical work and training workshops he has elucidated several types of Transference Neurosis. He considers Transference Neurosis to be a morbid process in psychotherapy and when present adds a destructive system on top of an already destructive, self-damaging masochistic character structure in a person suffering from early trauma and fusion, often combined with an intergenerational transfer of neurosis. In the training workshops he has devised variations in the therapeutic process and has applied it to the training setting to address the various forms of Transference Neurosis. His work in this endeavor is ongoing and he continues to present his results in his Audio-Visual symposia. He has repeatedly demonstrated that Transference Neurosis, though complex and difficult, can be a reversible process. I wish to acknowledge my heartfelt gratitude to Dr. Davanloo for allowing me to participate in this process with him over these past two and a half decades. All of the ideas, concepts and principles presented in this chapter are his discoveries. He has generously shared them over the years and encouraged me to synthesize them for others and for myself by presenting at his annual symposia and by writing this chapter. What is clear to me at this point, is that rather than a term ready for abandonment or retirement, Transference Neurosis is a destructive force that needs to be reckoned with for successful psychotherapy and for human growth. Fortunately, Davanloo has alerted us to the role it plays in our most difficult cases and in ourselves and has pointed the way for us towards reversing and resolving this destructive process.

REFERENCES

Alexander, F. and French, T.E. (1980) (first published 1946), *Psychoanalytic therapy: principles and application*, Lincoln: University of Nebraska Press.

Beeber, A. (1999a). The perpetrator of the unconscious in Davanloo's new metapsychology. Part I: Review of classic psychoanalytic concepts. *International Journal of Intensive Short-Term Dynamic Psychotherapy*, 13, 151-157.

Beeber, A. (1999b). The perpetrator of the unconscious in Davanloo's new metapsychology. Part II: Comparison of the perpetrator to classic psychoanalytic concepts. *International Journal of Intensive Short-Term Dynamic Psychotherapy*, 13, 159-176.

Beeber, A. (1999c). The perpetrator of the unconscious in Davanloo's new metapsychology. Part III: Specifics of Davanloo's technique. *International Journal of Intensive Short-Term Dynamic Psychotherapy*, 13, 177-189.

Beeber, A.R. (2016).

Brenner, C. (1982) *The mind in conflict*. New York: International Universities Press.

Chessick, R.D. (2002). Psychoanalytic peregrinations I: Transference and transference neurosis revisited. *Journal of the American Academy of Psychoanalysis*, 30(1), 83-97.

Cooper, A.M. (1987) The transference neurosis: A concept ready for retirement. *Psychoanalytic Inquiry*, 7:4, 569-585.

Davanloo, H. (1975) Proceedings of the First International Symposium and Workshop on Short-Term Dynamic Psychotherapy, Montreal, Canada. March 19-22.

Davanloo, H. (19776) Proceedings of the Second International Symposium and Workshops on Short-Term Dynamic Psychotherapy, Montreal, Canada. March 29-April 3.

Davanloo, H. (1977) Proceedings of the Third International Symposium and Workshops on Short-Term Dynamic Psychotherapy, Century Plaza, Los Angeles, California. November 9-13.

Davanloo, H. (Ed.) (1980a). *Short-term dynamic psychotherapy.* New York: J. Aronson.

Davanloo, H. (1980). A method of short-term dynamic psychotherapy. In: H. Davanloo (Ed.) *Short-term dynamic psychotherapy* (pp. 43-71). New York: J. Aronson.

Davanloo, H. (1990a). Clinical manifestations of super-ego pathology, Part I. In: *Unlocking the unconscious: Selected papers of Habib Davanloo, MD* (pp. 163-192). Chichester, England: Wiley (Reprinted from *International Journal of Short-Term Psychotherapy*, 2 (4)(1987), 225-254.

Davanloo, H. (1990b). Clinical manifestations of super-ego pathology, Part II. The resistance of the superego and the liberation of the paralyzed ego. In: *Unlocking the unconscious: Selected papers of Habib Davanloo, MD* (pp. 193-216) (Reprinted from *International Journal of Short-Term Psychotherapy*, 3(1), (1988) 1-24.

Davanloo, H. (1991-1993) Syracuse Core Training Program in Davanloo's Intensive Short-Term Dynamic Psychotherapy, Syracuse, NY.

Davanloo, H. (1993, 1997-2005) Montreal Core Training Program in Davanloo's Intensive Short-Term Dynamic Psychotherapy, Montreal, QC, CA.

Davanloo, H. (2000a). Intensive short-term dynamic psychotherapy Spectrum of psychoneurotic disorders. *Intensive short-term dynamic psychotherapy: Selected papers of Habib Davanloo, MD.* (p. 4) Chichester, England: Wiley (Reprinted from *International Journal of Short-Term Psychotherapy*, 10(3/4) (1995), 121-155.

Davanloo, H. (2000b). Intensive short-term dynamic psychotherapy Technique of partial and major unlocking of the unconscious with a highly resistant patient. Part I Partial unlocking In: *Intensive short-term dynamic psychotherapy: Selected papers of Habib Davanloo, MD.* (p. 47) Chichester, England: Wiley (Reprinted from *International Journal of Short-Term Psychotherapy*, 10(3/4) (1995), 157-181.

Davanloo, H. (2001) Intensive short-term dynamic psychotherapy: Extended major direct access to the unconscious. *European Psychotherapy*, 2 (2) 25-70.

Davanloo, H. (2005). Intensive Short-Term Dynamic Psychotherapy. In: *Kaplan and Sadock's comprehensive textbook of psychiatry* (8th ed., pp. 2628-2652). Philadelphia, Pa. Lippincott Williams and Wilkins.

Davanloo, H. (2007-2015). Proceedings of the 28th-36th Annual Audio Visual Symposia in the Mobilization of the Unconscious and Davanloo's Intensive Short-Term Dynamic Psychotherapy. Montreal, Canada.

Davanloo, H. (2007-2016). Proceedings of the Montreal Closed-Circuit Experiential Training Workshops in the Mobilization of the Unconscious and Davanloo's Intensive Short-Term Dynamic Psychotherapy. Montreal, Canada.

Davanloo, H. (2009). Proceedings of the 30th Annual Audiovisual Immersion Course on Technique of the Process of Working Through: The Revolutionary Discovery of Fusion of Primitive Murderous Rage and Guilt in Highly Resistant Patients and the Technique of De-Fusion: Fusion of Primitive Murderous Rage and Sexuality and the Technique of De-Fusion. Montreal, Canada. October 5-10.

Davanloo, H. (2010). Proceedings of the 31st Annual Audiovisual Immersion Course on the Metapsychology of the Unconscious: The Revolutionary Discovery of the Technique of Total Removal of Resistance. Montreal, Canada. October 4-9.

Davanloo, H. (2011). Proceedings of the 32nd Annual Audiovisual Immersion Course on the Metapsychology of the Unconscious: An Extensive Audiovisual Exploration. Montreal, Canada. October 3-8.

Davanloo, H. (2012). Proceedings of the 33rd Annual Audiovisual Immersion Course on the Metapsychology of the Unconscious: An Extensive Exploration of the Dynamic Unconscious. Montreal, Canada. October 1-5.

Davanloo, H. (2013). Proceedings of the 34th Annual Audiovisual Symposium on the Metapsychology of the Unconscious: An Extensive Exploration of the Dynamic Unconscious. Montreal, Canada. October 7-11.

Davanloo, H. (2014). Proceedings of the 35th International Audiovisual Symposium on the Science of the Metapsychology of the Unconscious: An Extensive Experiential Clinical Audio-Visual Exploration of the Dynamic Unconscious. Montreal, Canada. October 6-10.

Davanloo, H. (2015). Proceedings of the 36th International Audiovisual Symposium on the Science of the Metapsychology of the Unconscious: Davanloo's Technique of Major Mobilization of the Unconscious; the Technique of Total Removal of Resistance; and Davanloo's Intensive Short-Term Dynamic Psychotherapy. Montreal, Canada. October 5-9.

Freud, S. (1905/19) Fragment of an analysis of a case of hysteria. In: *The standard edition of the complete psychological works of Sigmund Freud* (Vol XII, pp. 99-108). Translated and edited by Strachey, J. London: Hogarth Press [for] the Institute of Psychoanalysis, 1991.

Freud, S. (1912) The dynamics of the transference. In: *The standard edition of the complete psychological works of Sigmund Freud* (Vol VII, pp. 1-22).

"Psychoanalytic Therapy: Principles and Application" was released in 1946 [4]. This detailed a psychodynamic approach that was both time limited and active. There was flexibility in the therapist's approach and the therapist was now transformed from a passive observer to an active participant in the therapeutic process. In this model, the therapist could work with and control the development of transference feelings in repsonse to the perceived therapeutic needs of the patient. This approach was initially met with some trepidation by those in the psychoanalytic community.

However, this change in focus led to a paradigm shift in the world of psychodynamic psychotherapy. Some psychoanlysts embraced the change of their roles and gladly became more active in the process. In this era of experimentation, therapists began to see the importance of not only managing but appropriately developing transference through the course of an interview. These therapists reported that in a group of carefully selected patients, more active, time-limited techniques could be employed to result in more robust clinical change.

In the process of independent work, four individuals devleoped their own models of brief dynamic psychotherapy. In the 1960s-1970s, they began to see the commonality of their approaches and worked together to develop symposia and congresses throughout the world. They aimed to discuss a more active, time limited approach towards dynamic psychotherapy. Each indivdual model will be reviewed briefly below.

MODELS OF BRIEF DYNAMIC PSYCHOTHERAPIES

David Malan worked at the Tavistock Institute under the direction of Michael Balint in the UK. Malan's Brief Psychotherapy was seen as interpretive nature [5]. His selection criteria included patients who had a single psychotherapeutic focus, were responsive to interpretation and had at least one other meaningful relationship. In addition, his patients were highly motivated and tended to have symptoms or disturbances of more recent onset. As such, he tended to avoid more highly resistant patients as they tended to be less motivated.

Peter Sifneos developed his Short-Term Anxiety-Provoking Psychotherapy at Harvard University [6]. Also known for rigid selection criteria with patient motivation being at the top of his list, he had the same population of less resistant patients as did Malan. Like Malan, he tended not to directly confront resistance. He also worked in the transference, focusing on underlying feelings—thereby creating anxiety. Also like Malan, he focused on patients who had a single, circumscribed problem.

Mann also worked in Boston and formulated his "Time-Limited Psychotherapy" [7]. In the initial evaluative interview, he sought to empathically understand the patient and summarized their "present and chronically endured pain" at the end of the session. Thereafter, he would set a time limit and commit to meet with the patient for 12 one hour sessions. This time limited focus was felt to result in maximum commitment and adherence to the process and the goals of therapy. But given this focus on a time limited therapy, several themes invariably arose—most notably attachment and loss. As such, these patients needed to be able to tolerate the resulting painful affect. They tended to be highly motivated and less resistant without any underlying characterological problems.

Davanloo developed the McGill Short-Term Psychotherapy Program with his colleagues at McGill University in Montreal, Canada. He has spent the last four decades refining his techniques. His therapy has been described as unique by both critics and supporters alike. Davanloo directly and actively engages with the patient to rapidly mobilize the twin factors which are the cornerstone of his technique: transference feelings and resistance.

Davanloo's unique understanding of the human unconscious has been called "the Metapsychology of the Unconscious." This chapter is devoted to an in-depth exploration of Davanloo's work. The goals will be threefold. First, the early work of Davanloo and his Metapsychology of the Unconscious will be reviewed. Secondly, we will review his newest training program which is called the Montreal Closed Circuit Training Program. Thirdly, we will review his newest discoveries, techniques and approaches—most of which have been disseminated through the Montreal Closed Circuit Training Program. These three goals will not be contained in three separate sections; rather important older and newer concepts will be interwoven throughout the text. New clinical vignettes will be added where possible to illustrate important concepts.

Davanloo's Approach to Training

As mentioned, Davanloo has developed his own unique understanding of the human unconscious which he refers to as the Metapsychology of the Unconscious. Before we explore this in detail, it is important to note several important aspects of Davanloo's research and teaching which have led him to arrive at his theories.

Davanloo firmly believed (and still believes) in the importance of video-technology in the training process. Early in his career, he pioneered the use of videotaping in dynamic therapy. Many therapists and analysts felt that the use of a video camera and microphone would be deleterious to the patient and to the development of a working alliance. However, Davanloo still obtains the informed, written consent for every patient that he videotapes. As such, he does not rely on process notes which he argues are subject to recall bias. In his earlier years as a supervisor, trainees were expected to show their work for not only Davanloo to see, but often for an audience of therapists/trainees to see. While this might initially provoke anxiety in the trainee (and the patient), it was expected that the trainee would work through this as supervision progresses. This is in keeping with a long history of allowing trainees to discover and work through any unconscious blocks they may have in providing therapy to their patients. It has long been assumed that this is beneficial not only to the trainee him or herself, but also to the patient—as better therapy should result from this process.

Davanloo's use of video-technology has resulted in many important and noteworthy elements. For one, Davanloo has a library of thousands of teaching tapes. In the absence of process notes, there is no debate about what has happened in the psychotherapy room. Videotapes, which contain important information on process and content are available for supervisor and trainee to watch--often repeatedly. With this comes a unique vantage point in to the unconscious. Both verbal and non-verbal cues can be witnessed, analyzed and understood. While the unconscious remains a complex entity in many patients, the use of video-technology has allowed Davanloo and his trainees to more accurately diagnose and dissect the process—many have argued that this dissection is critical to Davanloo's work. Some have anecdotally described the dissection as having a surgical precision.

Secondly, the use of video technology has led to an atmosphere of openness in Davanloo's process. Trainees cannot hide from the reality of their work. There is a vulnerability associated with showing one's work and inviting others to comment on and scrutinize it. It is important to note that trainees are not coerced in to this training format. Indeed, they are made aware of the format and process and either seek out and consent to it or not. This openness tends to mobilize emotions in the trainees. Many of these emotions are mobilized from the unconscious. What results is a unique training model in which trainees cannot avoid their emotions. Either they pledge to an atmosphere of honesty and integrity; in which they choose to face and experience their unconscious emotions at their fullest intensity, or they do not.

Davanloo repeatedly emphasizes the participants' will, choice and voluntary consent in engaging in the training process.

Davanloo's Metapsychology of the Unconscious

At this time, it is necessary to review some important basic concepts of the Metapsychology of the Unconscious. It should be noted that Davanloo did not arrive at his discoveries in an instantaneous fashion. Rather, he spent countless hours repeatedly watching his own (and his trainees') videotapes. By carefully analyzing the process (and by inviting others to do so at his symposia throughout the decades) he came to appreciate which interventions worked and which did not [8]. He was able to theorize around his work in order to develop the model of the unconscious which will be outlined below.

The Pathogenic Core of the Unconscious

Davanloo's Metapsychology of the unconscious is often best understood in narrative form. At the beginning of the narrative is a human being's love and attachment to important early childhood figures known as genetic figures. Usually these figures are parents, grandparents, and/or siblings. But they can be any important early childhood figures. Like Bowlby [9], Davanloo believes that love and attachment to these early genetic figures is essential to the healthy psychological development of any child. If this love or attachment is disrupted, then it causes psychological damage to the child. While this may seem fairly intuitive in nature, Davanloo has gone on to theorize the exact constellation of unconscious phenomena which results from the disruption of love and attachment to early genetic figures.

Following disruption of the attachment, an individual suffers the pain of this trauma. Again, Davanloo has defined the unconscious sequelae of such pain. He has summarized the layers of the pain in a diagram. See Figure 1 below.

Firstly, the patient develops murderous rage towards the genetic figure. Davanloo has often described this murderous rage as lying on a spectrum. On one hand, it can be purely murderous in nature. On the other side of the spectrum it can have primitive qualities and be torturous in nature. More recently, he has described some patients as having not only primitive, murderous torturous rage but pure sadism towards genetic figures. This has been discussed more recently in his Closed Circuit Training Program [10] which will be reviewed below. It is important to note that this murderous rage is of such an intense quality that it remains unconscious in most patients—often until they pursue therapy.

Often associated with the murderous rage are sexual feelings. These are often fused together. Fusion has been a more recent concept in Davaloo's work and will also be reviewed in further detail below. Essentially, when some patients experience murderous rage towards the therapist, they simultaneously experience sexual feelings. It is important to note that while these may be directed towards the therapist in the moment that the patient feels the murderous impulse, the patient in no way develops an ongoing, sustained sexual attraction to the therapist. The latter would be more in keeping with a transference neurosis which commonly develops in traditional psychoanalysis. While the development of transference neurosis was commonplace in psychoanalysis, Davanloo avoids it all costs in his work. For further information on this, see the section on transference neurosis below.

Following the experience of this intense murderous rage (with or without sexual feelings), the patient goes on to experience guilt. It is important to note that the experience of guilt is not a cognitive one. The patient has the true physical experience of this emotion. The physical experience of guilt is fairly unique to Davanloo's work. It will be reviewed in more detail under the section on the neurobiological pathway below. Essentially, guilt involves a painful constriction of the muscles of the chest and larynx. It comes in waves. Participants in Davanloo's program have anecdotally reported this experience as one of the most painful physical sensations that they have ever had. However, the success of the process depends on several factors – one of which is the patient's successful, affective experience of guilt. Much analysis of videotapes/DVDs in this work has focused on whether or not the patient's experience is consistent with true guilt or grief.

The unconscious guilt may be associated with affect laden grief feelings. Grief is similar to guilt in that it comes in waves. However it is not associated with the same painful constriction of the muscles of the upper airway, chest and larynx. While it is painful to experience, it is not as painful as the experience of unconscious guilt—which is qualitatively a much different experience. While grief can consist of waves of painful feelings associated with tearfulness, it is not associated with the same degree of painful muscular contraction. In addition, while grief may consist of sadness, it is not associated with the same intense sorrow and regret for the actions that the patient has (unconsciously) committed.

Because of this constellation of very painful unconscious emotions, the patient develops major resistance. When the painful unconscious emotions are extremely intense, the patient develops character resistance. Davanloo has coined the very important term, "Resistance Against Emotional Closeness." This refers to the patient's specific character resistance of not allowing him or herself to have true emotional closeness and intimacy in life. While this term is not captured in DSM 5 [11] and does not, in and of itself, connote a personality or character disorder, it does refer to a very widespread phenomenon that is seen in clinical and community populations throughout the world. It is a very common character resistance in therapists who seek out training with Davanloo and participate in the Montreal Closed Circuit Training Program.

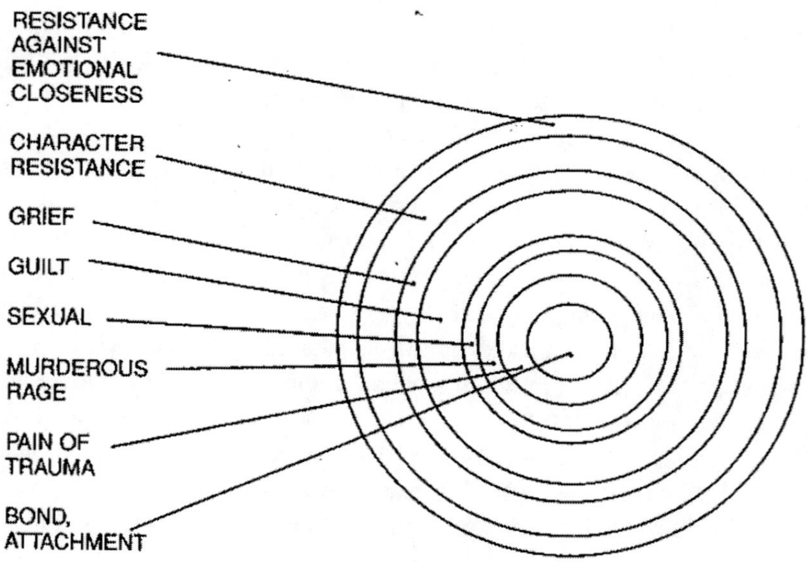

Figure 1. The Pathogenic Core of the Unconscious (Davanloo, 2000).

The pathogenic core of the unconscious is a very helpful schematic approach at understanding the unconscious forces which lie at the heart of the patient's character and symptom disturbances. Anecdotally, many participants in the Montreal Closed Circuit Training Program have commented on Davanloo's unique ability to use the pathogenic core to provide an etiological formulation of the patients and participants he works with. Simply put, the etiological formulation is the articulated understanding of why a patient presents a certain way at a certain time. Understanding the exact psychodynamics of early attachment and loss provides an invaluable guide to understanding the present day reality, circumstances, and constellation of symptoms that a patient presents with.

In his more recent work, Davanloo has talked about the concept of "fusion." This is directly related to the pathogenic core of the unconscious and will be reviewed in a separate section below.

The Neurobiological Pathway

The neurobiological pathway is an important construct which is central to Davanloo's metapsychology of the unconscious. The neurobiological pathway is a clearly outlined theory on how the unconscious intersects with the human body in a physiological manner. At the present time, Davanloo has described the neurobiological pathways of murderous rage, sexuality, guilt and memory. Each of these will be reviewed below and are summarized in Figure 2.

Davanloo's technical approach to working with the patient's unconscious is referred to as the central dynamic sequence and will be outlined below. As Davanloo works with the patient using this series of steps, the patient develops both resistance and transference feelings. Both resistance and transference feelings have been referred to as the "Twin Factors" and are an important cornerstone of the technique as mentioned. They also will be reviewed in more detail below.

To summarize, as one applies the central dynamic sequence and monitors the patient for the development of resistance and transference feelings, one can observe the patient's verbal and non-verbal communication for the presence of both unconscious anxiety and unconscious emotions. Davanloo does not believe that these feelings have only cognitive (or intellectual concomitants). Rather he believes that unconscious anxiety and emotions have distinct physiological concomitants that are largely similar (albeit expressed in slightly different ways) across various patient populations.

The neurobiological pathway of unconscious anxiety will be reviewed in more detail in the section below called "The Discharge Patterns of Unconscious Anxiety." Suffice to say, there are various ways that unconscious anxiety can be experienced by a patient and clinically manifested in an interview.

To start with, Davanloo noticed early on that his active and relentless approach (which starts with a phase of inquiry that later segues into various other steps of the central dynamic sequence) often resulted in the later development of murderous rage. Often patients use tactical defenses to either deny, minimalize or negate the presence of this murderous rage. However, when these tactical defenses are dealt with or dismissed by the therapist, these patients often experience the true sensation of their physiological murderous rage. Often, it is described as a "fireball" or as a "volcano." It tends to start in the lower abdomen/pelvis and has the propensity to move upwards and outwards. In this sense, it has a tendency to want to launch out and attack. While slightly different in presentation, this experience has been remarkably similar amongst patients of different genders, backgrounds, cultures and ethnicities. Depending on the degree of murderous rage it can be mild or more severe. It can have primitive and tortuous qualities. In some, more highly damage patients, it can only be considered as pure sadism. This phenomenon has been described more recently by Davanloo in his Montreal Closed Circuit Training Program [12]. Earlier in his career, Davanloo described patients who were less damaged and fell on the left side of the spectrum of psychoneurosis (this will be reviewed in detail below). These healthier, less damaged patients often had circumscribed problems or a single focus. Davanloo found that many of these patients had minimal, if any murderous rage in their unconscious. They were often highly responsive. But many of the professional therapists he works with today have highly primitive, tortuous, murderous rage and sadism in their unconscious. These patients are far more complicated and far more resistant to therapy.

Next, is the neurobiological pathway of guilt. As discussed in the section on the pathogenic core of the unconscious, Davanloo describes guilt as both an affective and physiological experience; rather than a cognitive one. It usually occurs after the patient has the full experience of the neurobiological pathway of murderous rage and the impulse to murder the therapist. However, it can occur after a patient experiences positive feelings towards the therapist as well. When the patient murders the therapist, the therapist usually tells the patient to focus on the image of the murdered body. While doing so, there is a very complex, yet replicable unconscious phenomenon. The unconscious transfers the visual image of the murdered therapist to a visual image of an important genetic figure which the patient has murdered. When this genetic figure becomes clear, the patient often experiences a profound feeling of guilt. As outlined above, this experience of guilt is one of the important therapeutic factors in Davanloo's technique—many would argue that it is indeed a curative factor. As also outlined, it is a uniquely painful feeling involving constriction of the muscles of the chest, larynx and upper airway. Sometimes, if the session has not gone as smoothly as planned, the patient can experience bronchospasm and/or coughing. Therefore, it is important for all therapists to have maximum supervision in the early stages of their practice.

More recently Davanloo has discussed the neurobiological pathway of memory. These discussions have occurred in the various Montreal Closed Circuit Training Program workshops as well as his Annual Metapsychology meetings in Montreal [10, 13]. When the neurobiological pathways of murderous rage/sadism and guilt are activated in a maximum fashion, the patient often reports the return of important memories that had hitherto been repressed. Usually, these memories are rich in vivid detail. Since they often occur at a time in the interview when the resistance is not present – or at least greatly diminished – they offer a rich communication about the patient's pathogenic core of the unconscious and how it relates to their ongoing life circumstances. They are of vast importance to the therapeutic process. Often, when these are offered, the therapist chooses to be silent, or at least to reflect on the content and meaning of these memories. It is very important not to introduce speculation at this point. Davanloo speaks in his workshops about following the "Trail of the Unconscious"[10]. Focusing on the rich visual details or the circumstances of the events is often enough to trigger the unconscious to provide further communication about the significance of the memory.

When the unconscious is sufficiently mobilized, each of the neurobiological pathways becomes mobilized. This is represented in the schematic diagram below.

The Discharge Patterns of Unconscious Anxiety

The use of video-technology in Davanloo's technique offers a unique opportunity to understand the content of what a patient says during an interview. It also offers a unique opportunity to visualize and understand the non-verbal communication of the patient. Davanloo, after viewing countless hours of videotapes in his early career, began to note the various ways that a patient's unconscious anxiety would manifest and discharge in response to his interventions. These discharge patterns of unconscious anxiety will be reviewed below:

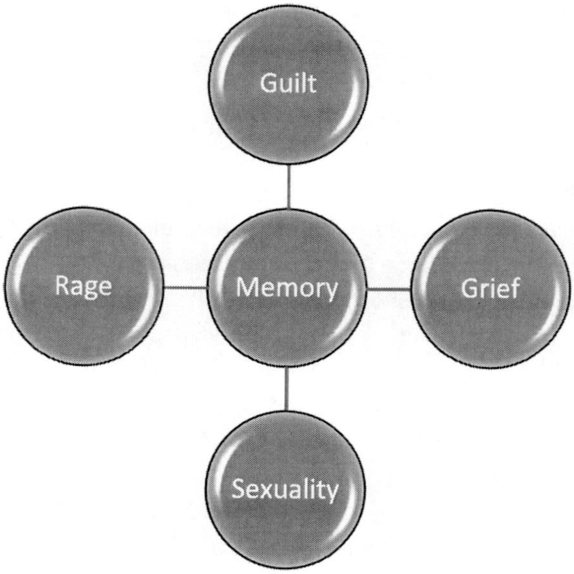

Figure 2. The Neurobiological Pathway [12].

1. The Striated Muscle Discharge Pattern

As Davanloo developed the steps of the central dynamic sequence (see below), he realized that some steps caused the patient to be more anxious. In healthier patients, who often had a single focus and circumscribed problem, the interventions of the central dynamic sequence resulted in a clear cut response. These patient would have activation of the striated muscles of their body. The therapist could visualize flexion and extension of the patient's thumbs, fingers and hands. This usually would progress to involve the intercostal muscles. These patients would often have sighing respirations in response to Davanloo's interventions.

Such patients would be far easier to monitor on videotapes. Even in rewinding and fast forwarding tapes, Davanloo and his participants could clearly visualize a patient sighing and clenching their hands. This lead to a very predictable response such that a patient's unconscious signaling system was easily visualized and monitored. Davanaloo was able to see which interventions were effective in such patients—leading to mobilization of further unconscious anxiety, transference feelings, and resistance – and which weren't.

2. The Smooth Muscle Discharge Pattern

While Davanloo was developing the central dynamic sequence, he noted another group of patients who were less easy to monitor. In these patients, there would often be an absence of clear cut striated muscle discharge. Instead of sighs and clenching hand movements, there would often be no visual signaling. Interestingly, these patients, sometimes reported other phenomena. When Davanloo inquired about their status and how they were doing, some reported abdominal pain or the urge to defecate. Others reported the onset of a headache. Davanloo concluded that these patients did not have the primary discharge pattern of striated muscle. Rather, he concluded that the patients did indeed have unconscious anxiety but it was discharged through the smooth muscles of the body rather than the striated muscles. Since the bowel/intestines and cerebral blood vessels have smooth muscle, patients with this type of discharge pattern can report gastrointestinal symptoms and/or headache.

3. Cognitive/Perceptual Disruption

Some patients did not have the above more clear-cut discharge pathways of unconscious anxiety. When Davanloo intiated the various steps in the central dynamic sequence, such patients did not have activation of either the striated muscles or the smooth muscles. Instead, they had disturbance in their cognitive and/or perceptual fields. For example, some of these patients became confused as the interview progressed—often when more challenging and affect laden zones were approached. Others dissociated and Davanloo came to know this only upon directly questioning the patients about what had happened in the preceding moments. Others experienced hallucinations—for example, hearing people screaming or seeing people being tortured. The patients who experienced cognitive/perceptual disruption tended to be more damaged than those who did not. They will be reviewed in detail below in the section on the spectrum of character fragility.

The Spectrum of Psychoneurotic Disorders

Again, after watching countless of hours of videtoapes, Davanloo came to see that patients presented in very different ways depending on their different make-ups and backgrounds. He described two spectra upon which patients could be classified. These are the spectrum of psychoneurotic disorders and the spectrum of character fragility. As a rule, those patients who fall on the spectrum of psychoneurosis tend to be less damaged and more responsive to therapy than the patients who fall on the spectrum of character fragility.

He defined 5 groups on the spectrum of psychoneurotic disorders [14]. The groups are as follows:

1. Extreme left on the spectrum
2. Mid-left side on the spectrum
3. Mid-spectrum
4. Mid-right side on the spectrum
5. Extreme right side on the spectrum

1. The extreme left side of the spectrum refers to patients who have some degree of psychoneurotic illness but they are the least damaged of all of the patients who fall on this spectrum. They tend to have a single focus of therapy, a tightly circumscribed problem and are highly responsive to therapy. Murderous rage is absent in the unconscious of these patients. As such, they have a very mild degree of resistance. They tend to have symptom disturbances only—such as a mild obsessional neurosis-- with no major character pathology.
2. The mid-left side of the spectrum includes patients who have a moderate degree of resistance. These patients do have murderous rage as well as guilt- and grief-laden feelings in the unconscious. They have diffuse symptom disturbances and the presence of at least some character disturbance. There is no single focus and Davanloo describes them as having a multifocal core neurotic structure.
3. Mid-spectrum patients, as the name would suggest, lie directly in the center of the spectrum and have a moderate to high degree of resistance. They suffer from character neurosis which often leads to their presenting for psychotherapy. The have unconscious murderous rage and guilt- and grief-laden feelings in the unconscious. Sexuality may be fused with their murderous rage. They have complicated pathology at the heart of the pathogenic core of the unconscious. They tend to have masochism in their unconscious as well.
4. The mid-right side of the spectrum refers to a group that is more highly resistant than the mid-spectrum patients. They tend to have highly complicated pathology at the core of their unconscious. They suffer from diffuse and often lifelong symptom and character disturbances. These patients have extensive primitive, murderous rage, guilt and grief towards multiple genetic figures in their

unconscious. Murderous rage and sexuality are extensively fused in the unconscious. Davanloo has coined the phrase, "The Perpetrator of the Unconscious" [15]. This refers to a patient's unconscious tendency to inflict suffering and destructiveness on not only him/herself but others around him/her as well. It is heavily involved in a patient's self-defeating and self-sabotaging patterns, tendencies and behaviors. It is fundamental in the metapsychology of masochism and is as a direct manifestation of the guilt's desire to inflict suffering as a form of punishment for the primitive murderous rage.

5. Extreme right side of the spectrum refers to that group which is most highly resistant on the psychoneurotic spectrum. These patients are those with an extreme degree of resistance. They have had lifelong, severe, symptom and character disturbances. They have highly primitive, tortuous, murderous rage in their unconscious. In his most recent training program, Davanloo refers to these patients as having "pure sadism" in the unconscious [10]. This is in relation to multiple genetic figures. As a result of this sadism, these patients have extensive guilt in their unconscious, a punitive superego and highly masochistic character traits. There is an extensive degree of fusion of the murderous rage and guilt in the unconscious of these patients. As a result, these patients are highly resistant, highly complicated and their character pathology is often extremely ego syntonic.

The Spectrum of Character Fragility

As indicated above, the spectrum of character fragility generally refers to a group of patients who have more complicated psychopathology in comparison to the group of patients who fall on the spectrum of psychoneurotic disorders. There can be mild, moderate and severe fragility. Mild fragility might refer to patients who do not dissociate/drift/hallucinate unless the central dynamic sequence visits some very painful zones in the unconscious. Severe character fragility might refer to those patients who present to the interview with dissociation/drifting/hallucinations in the absence of any therapist intervention. Moderate fragility lies somewhere in between.

Overall, these patients do not have the capacity to tolerate anxiety and extremely painful feelings. As a result, they do not have the capacity to withstand the impact of their own unconscious during a single interview. Because of this, Davanloo made several modifications of his technique and adopted a "graded approach" to working with these patients. Using this approach, the therapist aims to create sufficient unconscious structural changes over time. With the development of these structural changes, the patient has a shift in how they experience and discharge anxiety. These patients begin to have less dissociation/drifting and perceptual experiences and begin to discharge their anxiety more in the striated muscles. The graded approach is a complicated one, has been reviewed in numerous symposia [16-18], and should not be practiced by those who have insufficient experience in the technique.

The Twin Factors of Transference Feelings and Resistance

Early on in his career, Davanloo began dissecting the therapeutic process in an effort to better understand the therapeutic factors which laid the foundation for success. He soon discovered that the cornerstone of his technique were the twin factors of transference feelings and resistance [19]. Specifically, the progress of the interview depended on the transference feelings that the patient developed towards the therapist and the degree of resistance that was generated in the patient. The therapist, therefore, would begin the interview by observing the status of any transference feelings or resistance that was already present. When absent, the therapist would search for these. The goal would be to scan the unconscious and focus on areas which increase both resistance and transference feelings. What resulted was an increased intensity of both feelings towards the therapist (as he or she focused on areas of unconscious conflict and pain) and resistance towards the therapist—in an effort to avoid experiencing these painful unconscious emotions. These two factors were initially described by Davanloo in the 1980s/1990s. He has more recently defined the intersection of these two factors (the Transference Component of the Resistance—or the TCR) as the most important therapeutic parameter which guides the process [20]. This will be reviewed in more detail below.

The Unconscious Therapeutic Alliance

Davanloo has received much criticism for his "rigorous, challenging clinical style" and "confrontational questioning and dogged use of transference"[21]. However, he has received much less attention for the development of the unconscious therapeutic alliance (or UTA). The unconscious therapeutic alliance is that part of the patient that wants to ally with the therapist, to be truthful with the therapist, and to face the most profound unconscious emotions, even if they are extremely painful [19]. As a result of Davanloo's active series of interventions, many patients report the development of warm, grateful, appreciative feelings. While there has been much focus on Davanloo's use of confrontation and challenge there has been far less attention paid to the warm, close and positive feelings that patients develop in Davanloo's therapy. Few of his critics are likely to comment on the patient's warm appreciation that a therapist will not accept what is on the surface but will work hard to help the patient examine what is below.

As the patient develops the sense that they are working with the therapist, the unconscious therapeutic alliance rises and strengthens in intensity. Transference feelings (which are often a mix of both warm, positive feelings and negative, murderous feelings—previously referred to as complex transference feelings) often strengthen in intensity. Once the UTA and transference feelings reach a critical threshold, the resistance weakens precipitously. When this happens, the patient has what is referred to as an "unlocking of the unconscious." This will be reviewed in further detail below. Some consider an unlocking of the unconscious to be synonymous with the term breakthrough in to the unconscious. When this occurs, feelings that had previously been unconscious enter the conscious zone; the patient experiences a unique catharsis related to these profound emotions and the communication that comes from the unconscious is not contaminated by resistance whatsoever.

The Transference Component of the Resistance

In recent training program workshops [13] and in his book chapter [20], Davanloo has discussed the importance of the intersection between the transference feelings and resistance—otherwise known as the TCR—as being the most important therapeutic parameter which guides the interview process. Developing the TCR is not an task—especially for a junior therapist who does not have adequate training and supervision [12]. Monitoring the TCR can also be challenging. Much of the training in Davanloo's Montreal Closed Circuit Training Program is spent focusing on the status of the TCR and any interventions a therapist can employ to further mobilize it. When the TCR fails to be mobilized—and this is often the case with junior therapists or those who have unconscious blocks—Davanloo and the group can offer ideas and suggestions on how to get the process back on track. It should be noted that this can be a very dynamic learning environment. A trainee can discover not only which patient factors prevent the optimum mobilization of the TCR but also which therapist factors limit the mobilization of the TCR. Feedback is often live and an interview can be interrupted so that a trainee can change his/her strategy and interventions. Group feedback often occurs after the live interview itself and/or after the interview DVD is watched. This type of focus on the process in general, and the status of the TCR specifically, creates a very rich learning environment in which participants can focus on competency based psychotherapy education. Given the current trend towards more competency based psychotherapy education [22], this environment is an ideal way for trainees to learn hands on advanced skills.

The Central Dynamic Sequence

Davanloo has operationalized his method of working with the unconscious. Unlike with traditional psychoanalysis, there is little in the way of passive listening in Davanloo's approach. Instead, Davanloo focuses on a steady balance between observing the patient (and being empathically attuned with their verbal and non-verbal cues) and taking an active and uncompromising stance with the patient's resistance.

It is important to note that Davanloo's approach is one of having the utmost respect for the patient but the utmost disrespect for the patient's resistance. Misalliance with the patient should never happen when this technique is used by a trained and experienced therapist.

His central dynamic sequence is one that he developed after watching hundreds of hours of videotaped interviews. It is important to note that each step of the central dynamic sequence need not be applied in order and that some steps may be omitted with some patients.

Essentially, there is flexibility in the approach. The therapist's task is to be empathically attuned with the patient and to follow the trail of the patient's unconscious; wherever that trail may lead. For this reason, there is no room for speculation nor the rote and mechanical application of the technique. Therapists need to be flexible and spontaneous when the patient's unconscious demands it.

A detailed review of scholarly articles on the central dynamic sequence exists [23-26]. What follows is a more abbreviated summary of the various steps.

The CDS consists of the following different phases: inquiry, pressure, challenge, transference resistance, direct access to the unconscious, systematic analysis of the transference, and dynamic exploration into the unconscious.

The therapist opens the interview with the phase of inquiry. If it is the initial psychodiagnostic interview with the patient, then the therapist might open with a question such as: "what is the problem that brings you here?" Despite the straightforward and direct nature of this question, many patients have problems with it. Some patients become vague about their problems or areas of disturbances that bring them to therapy. Often the therapist has to pursue this fundamental issue; not only for securing the therapeutic goals and contract but also because of the necessary implications on the patient's resistance. The therapist cannot tolerate vagueness, or imprecision (which are often just minor defences labelled as tactical defences). The therapist must engage the patient in openly declaring an active focus of therapy. Getting the patient to do often directly addresses that patient's ambivalence. As such, the phase of inquiry often activates unconscious emotions in the patient and quickly becomes dynamic in nature. Hence the term, dynamic inquiry.

Early on, the therapist often finds him or herself in a situation of needing to apply pressure for specificity or clarity. The phase of pressure simply refers to this systematic application. The therapist may ask the patient for more details about an event, for example. Alternatively, the therapist may ask the patient to simply be clear and less vague. If the therapist asks the patient for more details on how s/he feels or experiences a feeling, then the therapist would be using the phase of pressure to feelings. Often these feelings are in the transference (phase of pressure to the avoided feelings in the transference). But they can also be outside of the transference and focused on other important figures in the patient's current life (The "C" in the Triangle of Person which will be reviewed below). At any rate, this systematic exploration and unwillingness to settle for the surface details is referred to at the phase of pressure. It can be essential in increasing both transference feelings and resistance – and is sometimes all that is needed in creating an optimum rise in the TCR.

Following this, the classical teaching of Davanloo is that the therapist would then possibly engage in the phase of challenge. It is important to note the evolution of the phase of challenge in Davanloo's research and teaching. In the early years of his career, the phase of challenge meant calling on the patient's defence. In this sense, if the therapist observed the patient using a certain defence at a certain stage of the interview, s/he might clearly label it. The following would be an example. A professional female therapist is interviewed in the Closed Circuit Training Program. The therapist asks her about her grandmother. More details about her case will be reviewed below. The following is a vignette from the initial interview [27].

Interviewer: You took a sigh. What she was like when she was explosive?

Interviewee: It's hard to remember it, but I know it happened so many times. One memory doesn't jump out.

Interviewer: What do you account for that your memory suddenly collapses?

Interviewee: (sigh)

Interviewer: How do you feel right now?

Interviewee: I'm feeling a bit anxious.

Here the patient, who is a professional therapist, states that she doesn't remember what it was like when her grandmother was explosive. The therapist sees this inability to remember as a manifestation of resistance. One of her grandmother's main character defenses was to go explosive so it does not make metapsychological sense that she would fail to remember just one instance of this. The therapist is applying the phase of challenge by stating: "What do you account for that your memory suddenly collapses?" He is speaking the truth as the patient's memory is collapsing. But this is a very clear comment which pointedly addresses the patient's defense—that she is repressing important information about the grandmother because her complex feelings towards this woman are too painful.

While this is reflective of challenge it is important to note that it is not the systematic application of the phase of challenge. Davanloo used this much more extensively in the earlier phases of his career. The systematic application of the phase of challenge is only used during the phase of transference resistance. This phrase "transference resistance" refers to that phase of the interview when the resistance has crystallized in the transference—this essentially means that the TCR has become sufficiently high so that the central dynamic sequence can be appropriately applied to achieve a breakthrough in to the unconscious.

In the last decade, Davanloo has focused much more on the head-on collision (HOC) which is part of the phase of challenge. The head-on collision is the therapist's attempt at blocking all forces that maintain the resistance. For further information on all of the steps of the head-on collision, please see Gottwick et al. [26]. The therapist, whilst performing a head-on collision, often addresses the patient's will, the therapeutic task, the resistance inside and possibly outside of the transference, and applies pressure for the patient to remove the resistance inside of the transference. The head-on collision can only be applied in the context of the transference; it is a very direct communication with the patient and Davanloo has described it as the most powerful of all of the interventions of the central dynamic sequence [13]. It should not be used lightly or at the wrong time in the interview, and it requires extensive training in order for it to be used appropriately. It also tends to mobilize the unconscious of the therapist and for this reason, many therapists often avoid it. That said, it is a powerful intervention which can create a massive rise in the TCR. When it is applied at the correct time in the therapy session, the outcome can be dramatic.

When the transference feelings and unconscious therapeutic alliance reach a critical point, the resistance weakens considerably. With this, we see an unlocking of the unconscious which will be reviewed in detail below. When this happens, both the patient and therapist have direct access to the unconscious. This means that important unconscious emotions are available to the patient to be experienced in a physiological way. The experience of these feelings is in no way cognitive. Indeed, much of Davanloo's work over the last decade involves reviewing videotaped interviews and determining to what degree the patient's emotional experience was cognitive compared to affective. Once there has been direct access to the unconscious, there is systematic analysis of the transference, and dynamic exploration into the unconscious. Usually the therapist applies multidimensional unconscious structural changes at this part of the interview. Since the unconscious is not contaminated or influenced by resistance in any way at this time, the phase of dynamic exploration offers important information for both therapist and patient. It should also be noted that interpretation has no role in this technique until after the unlocking of the unconscious occurs.

The Unlocking of the Unconscious

Davanloo has written extensively on the unlocking of the unconscious [14]. He has classified four major types of unlockings below:

1. Partial unlocking of the unconscious
2. Major unlocking of the unconscious
3. Extended major unlocking of the unconscious
4. Extended, multiple major unlocking of the unconscious

Essentially, the degree of unlocking of the unconscious is determined by the degree to which the transference feelings and unconscious therapeutic alliance dominate the resistance. In addition, the higher the rise in the TCR, the more likely the resistance is to be dominated by transference feelings and unconscious therapeutic alliance.

The partial and major unlocking can be applied using Davanloo's standard technique of IS-TDP. However, the extended major, and extended, multiple major unlockings are only done in Davanloo's mobilization technique. This has been mastered by him and taught in the Montreal Closed Circuit Training Program which will be reviewed now.

The Montreal Closed Circuit Training Program

Davanloo's two books [14, 19] provide extremely in depth knowledge to anyone who is attempting to learn his technique. However, they do not provide the most current teaching on Davanloo's latest research findings and technical interventions. Since 2008, Davanloo has offered a unique training program. Therapists from around the world have applied to and been accepted in to this program. It involves a very unique experiential component; therapists have live, videotaped interviews with one another. Sometimes, Davanloo interviews participants himself. DVDs are then reviewed and analyzed repeatedly. What results is a number of phenomena:

1. There is a unique individual experiential component.
2. There is a unique group experiential component.
3. Important group dynamics such as universality, cohesion and instillation of hope come in to play [28].
4. The use of video-technology greatly reduces subjective bias as to what has transpired in the therapy session. Rather than attempts at recall and interpretation, there is direct evidence of the verbal and non-verbal communication of both patient and therapist.
5. As such, there is a tremendous focus on competency based psychotherapy education, which is in keeping with moves towards

teaching, assessing and evaluating skills; rather than focusing on knowledge acquisition alone.

The above factors result in a powerful training environment. While the exact number of blocks has varied from year to year, there is usually 3-5 blocks lasting for 5-6 days each. Participants are expected to fully immerse themselves in the training that is offered. It should be noted that this program, itself, offers only training and not treatment. Some participants in the Montreal Closed Circuit Training Program have sought out private treatment with Davanloo outside of this program. So there is often confusion about the nature of what occurs in the training program itself. At any rate, the correct nomenclature for participants in the program is not patient and therapist; rather it is interviewer and interviewee. Further details of the format of the Montreal Closed Circuit have been published elsewhere [27, 29, 30].

Some have criticized the Montreal Closed Circuit Training Program as being unconventional and as having [31] ethical concerns. It should be noted that this training program is just that—a training program. Participants enter this training program because they have sought out further education which will enable them to uncover any unconscious blocks which limit them as a therapist. There is written, informed consent for each participant. Participants are not obliged to participate if they do not wish to do so. While some have been invigorated by the process and have sought out private therapy with Davanloo, this has occurred in a minority of participants. As such, in a training program, participants can make a choice—they can choose to have training which will allow them to access and experience their unconscious feelings and resistance—or not. While some may express ethical concerns about participants interviewing one another, it should be noted that this has been a longstanding tradition. Trainees in psychotherapy have often undergone therapy with supervisors and have often revealed personal material in group formats with other trainees [32]. These concepts are not new. Indeed, the principles behind them—that a trainee would want to experience and understand that which limits him/her as a human being and a clinician—have been much cherished by those in the profession.

It is in the context of this unique, experiential training program, that Davanloo has developed and refined a number of new theories of his Metapsychology of the unconscious. The following sections will review some of these principles in further detail.

The Transference Neurosis

Freud believed that the development of the transference neurosis was an important aspect of psychoanalysis [33]. He felt that the development of the transference neurosis allowed, after careful analysis, both patient and therapist to better understand and work through the original neurosis. Freud argued that the transference neurosis was the "latest creation of the disease"[34]. In this sense, Freud saw the transference neurosis as a manifestation of the neurosis, rather than a manifestation of the treatment.

Davanloo takes a much different position. While he has not recently published on the transference neurosis, it has occupied a central position in his research and teaching in the last 5-10 years [10]. Davnaloo believes that the transference neurosis is not necessarily the development of the disease. The natural history of psychoneurosis is such that developing a transference neurosis is neither necessary nor normal. Davanloo would argue that the development of the transference neurosis is a manifestation of the treatment process. Specifically, the manifestation of a treatment process gone gravely awry. In Davanloo's work, there is not tolerance, whatsoever, for its development. This concept deserves further examination.

Davanloo believes that there are many different types of transference neuroses. His views on intergenerational transference neurosis and multi-dimensional intergenerational transference neurosis are fairly advanced and complex. While detailed examination of each is beyond the scope of this brief review, we will focus on three more basic and broad categories of the transference neurosis as below:

1. Transference neuroses that arise from treatment.
2. Transference neuroses that arise from training.
3. Transference neuroses that arise from professional practice.

The basic metapsychology of the first type of transference neurosis (which arises from treatment) is probably the easiest to understand. Davanloo speculates that transference neuroses develop in those individuals who have had treatment in which the TCR was too low to result in any major type of mobilization. Often, participants in the Montreal Closed Circuit Training Program present to the program having had previous treatment outside of the program. Often this outside treatment occurs with highly trained and experienced ISTDP therapists. As well it can occur with individuals who have very little direct supervision and training. In this latter situation, there are often no real unlockings of the unconscious. With a low TCR (which remains low throughout the course of therapy), there is fertile ground for the development of a transference neurosis towards the professional who provided therapy. Often such a transference neurosis revolves around certain ideations and feelings. The patient who developed the transference neurosis may have idealization of the former therapist and believe that s/he is infallible and providing stellar therapy.

The second type of transference neurosis results from the training programs individual therapists are exposed to. This might be a psychiatry residency, or various other graduate programs (psychology, social work, nursing, other medical fields). Often, individuals who supervise such trainees do not do so in an ethical fashion. Many of these supervisors have access to psychopathy in their own characters. Some abuse their positions of powers and degrade and disrespect the trainees. In this context, when trainees are put in to positions of submission to such supervision, there is, once again, fertile ground for development of a transference neurosis.

The third type of transference neurosis results from an individual therapist's work environment. In many academic and public settings, professional therapists are expected to assume large caseloads of often very complex patients. With this, the therapist becomes exposed to a large degree of character pathology in their patient population. This is not without risk. When working with such patients, it is possible that the therapist will be dramatically influenced by this work. Many therapists will report such work as exhausting. However, little research has been done to see how this work influences the therapist's own unconscious. Davanloo believes that such work—with many complex patients each of whom have a complex unconscious—leads to damage to the therapist's unconscious defensive organization. When this occurs, a variety of different phenomena can occur. The therapist can become symptomatic or develop character disturbances.

In the last 1-2 years, Davanloo has been working towards understanding exactly what gets "transferred" in a transference neurosis. Is it the individual's (therapist, patient or supervisor's) pathogenic core? Or is it there a transfer of the unconscious defensive organization? Or is it something else? The answer to this question is not yet clear but it remains an active focus of Davanloo's work.

To explore this concept further, a vignette will be explored. The case is the same one that was discussed earlier. The interviewee was a participant of the Montreal Closed Circuit Training Program. Her initial two interviews were published elsewhere [27, 35]. What follows is a vignette from her third interview which was originally published in another journal [30].

Her demographic details have been camouflaged so as to not reveal her identity. She is a 55 year old professional therapist who lives in Europe with her husband and children. She arrived at the Montreal Closed Circuit Training Program having had previous therapy with another individual. This therapy was not supervised but that therapist had previous training in ISTDP. The therapy spanned from 2004-2007 and consisted of three hour block sessions occurring about every 1-2 months. The patient had approximately 55 hours of therapy.

The patient had sought therapy for migraine headaches and mild relationship difficulties at that time. However, in 2007 she concluded that the therapy was no longer benefitting her and she terminated it.

She presented to the Montreal Closed Circuit Training Program initially in 2008. She had been interviewed by a number of other participants during various blocks. In 2012, she became acutely symptomatic with insomnia. She was able to identify that her main issue was intense anxiety which was focused on not getting to and staying asleep at night. She was interviewed in the Montreal Closed Circuit Training Program twice in July of 2012. During this time, she had intense breakthroughs to her grandmother. Her grandmother was an intensely stubborn yet loving woman who worked very hard during the Great Depression to provide for her family—including the patient's mother. She was referred to as "the Queen Bee" of the family. Everyone was compliant to her every wish and demand. The patient had a complicated relationship with her, but this never came up in any way during her previous therapy.

She has intense feelings towards her previous therapist. During the actual therapy with him, she had intense idealization of his work. As a therapist herself, she was able to identify this idealization as part of a transference neurosis. During her previous therapy, her breakthroughs focused mostly on her father. Her mother came up less often and her grandmother did not come up at all. During subsequent interviews in the Montreal Closed Circuit Training Program, it appeared that the original neurosis centered on her mother and grandmother. More specifically, at the pathogenic core of her unconscious, was a profoundly loving relationship with these very important, yet damaged, figures. What exactly was "transferred" in her transference neurosis with the previous therapist was unknown. But the patient had intense rage towards this figure. This will be outlined in the vignette below.

Interviewer: You see, again, the same principle: honesty, hmmm? That we face with everything with honesty. We really experience what we feel. That is the principle of life, isn't it?

Interviewee: I accept that.

Interviewer: You see you have a lot of feelings when you are not able to stand up in your interpersonal relationships. You see you have a lot of feelings about this therapy that you had because in a sense you allowed yourself to be walked all over. You have a lot of feeling.

Interviewee: I do.

Interviewer: Because you don't like to be walked over.

Interviewee: I hate it.

Interviewer: Because, next to you, it is your mother who went to a disaster in her life. So, you see you have that feeling.

Interviewee: I hate going catatonic. I hate that part of myself.

Interviewer: You say you hate to go catatonic.

Interviewee: But I do.

Interviewer: You do.

Interviewee: I do.

Interviewer: How do you feel right now? You took a sigh. How do you feel right now? Again, on the same principle, how do you experience this? See you are holding on this...

Interviewee: There is a rage building now.

Interviewer: It's building.

Interviewee: Yes. But it's not at its fullest intensity.

Interviewer: That, by itself, says something. The rage wants to build up, but you fight it. You don't want to be honest. Why don't you want to be honest?

Here the therapist is focusing on basic truths which are painful for the patient. This stirs up a lot of unconscious emotion in the patient. On one hand, the therapist begins the interview by focusing on the basic principle of honesty. The patient is an honest individual and she knows that there is no room for vagueness in the process. She adheres to this principle. But on the other hand the therapist addresses a basic character defence that the patient has used time and time again in her life. She has, in a sense, allowed many people to "walk all over her" in her interpersonal relationships in life. She knows that in many relationships she has gone “catatonic.” This creates tremendous unconscious feelings in the patient.

She acknowledges that she has this character trait/defence in many relationships. But it is extremely ego dystonic for her. The therapist states, “next to you, it is your mother who went to a disaster in her life.” This creates both positive and negative feelings in relationship to her mother. She has loving feelings towards her mother who was essentially a warm and affectionate human being. But she also has rage (and sadism) towards this individual who went catatonic in her own relationship with her mother (the patient’s grandmother).

While it seems like the therapist is working outside of the transference right now, he is actually working very powerfully in the transference. His examination of these issues is not only accurate it is relentless. The patient has complex feelings about his interventions. On one hand, she is deeply appreciative that the therapist (or any human being) would be so direct and relentless in pursuing her attachment and emotions towards her important genetic figures. On the other hand, her emotions towards these individuals are deeply painful and she would like to avoid experiencing them at all costs. But she instinctively knows that experiencing these feelings will be uniquely liberating for her and will heal her relationships with these family members. The part of her that wishes to avoid experiencing her emotions is reflective of her resistance. The part of her that wishes to have the liberating experience of her emotions is reflective of the unconscious therapeutic alliance that she has jointly created with the therapist.

The net result of these interventions is that there is an optimum mobilization of the Transference Component of the Resistance (or TCR). The interviewer knows that he has the “green light” to pursue the patient’s feelings towards him. She declares that she has a rage towards him and this signifies optimum mobilization of the neurobiological pathway of murderous rage in the transference. For the full transcript of the interview and detailed commentary on what transpired therein, see [30].

Fusion

Another important concept that Davanloo has developed in the last 5-10 years is the metapsychological notion of fusion. In order to understand this concept, the pathogenic core of the unconscious must be revisited.

In a normal healthy child/adult, unconscious emotions remain as distinct columns of feelings. They can be experienced in accordance with normal life events. In an individual who has psychoneurotic illness, the unconscious feelings do not remain in distinct columns in the unconscious. Rather they become fused or stuck to one another. They are not easily accessed by both patient and therapist. For example, murderous rage may be fused with guilt, or murderous rage may be fused with sexualized feelings. At any rate, the job becomes more complex for the therapist, as the feelings are not easy to access.

In these cases, patients can be completely unfamiliar with the experience of the neurobiological pathways of murderous rage and guilt. The therapist's job is to apply the central dynamic sequence in accordance with the patient's needs by following the "trail of the patient's unconscious" [13]. In doing so, s/he will facilitate the de-fusion of the unconscious emotions and the patient will have easier access to them. The age at which the pain of the trauma occurs is essential. Like many others [36], Davanloo believes that the earlier the age that the bond is disrupted, the greater the fusion.

Much of Davanloo's work in the Montreal Closed Circuit Training Program has been centered on working with highly resistant professional therapists. Like many resistant patients who fall on the mid-right and extreme right side of the spectrum, there is fusion which has occurred at an early age. Because of the complexities involved, the use of video-technology has been extremely helpful in understanding which interventions are most important in accessing the unconscious.

Multi-Dimensional Unconscious Structural Changes

Another important focus of Davanloo's more recent work has been the application of multi-dimensional unconscious structural changes (MUSC). What follows is a brief definition of MUSC and a discussion of their importance. A vignette will show how they were implemented in the fourth interview of the above patient in the Montreal Closed Circuit Training Program. For more detailed reading on this interview, see [37, 38].

MUSC are interventions that a therapist applies regardless of the stage of the central dynamic sequence. Some therapists apply them only after the unlocking of the unconscious and the breakthrough of murderous rage and guilt. However, they should be applied throughout the interview regardless of the stage the therapist and patient are in.

MUSC serve to allow the patient to make conscious sense of the unconscious experiences which occur in the session. While this definition may be simplistic and reductionistic to more senior therapists in the technique, it is a useful guide to help more junior clinicians best understand the multi-faceted and wide ranging scope of these interventions.

Simply put, MUSC are used to solidify the therapeutic task, to acquaint the patient with his/her resistance and to highlight the possibility for change [38]. Moment by moment, the therapist is constantly evaluating the status of the patient's unconscious and what is needed at that stage of the interview. Each verbal and non-verbal communication offers the therapist important information about the state of the patient's defense, anxiety and impulse—this Triangle of Conflict was first discussed by Ezriel [39]. Essentially, an individual has an unconscious impulse—this may be murderous in nature or it could be the impulse to experience loving and positive feelings towards an individual. Because of the unacceptable nature of the impulse, the patient defends against it—hence another corner of the triangle is represented by defense. Because of this underlying defended impulse, the individual develops anxiety. See Figure 3 below for a depiction of the Triangle of Conflict.

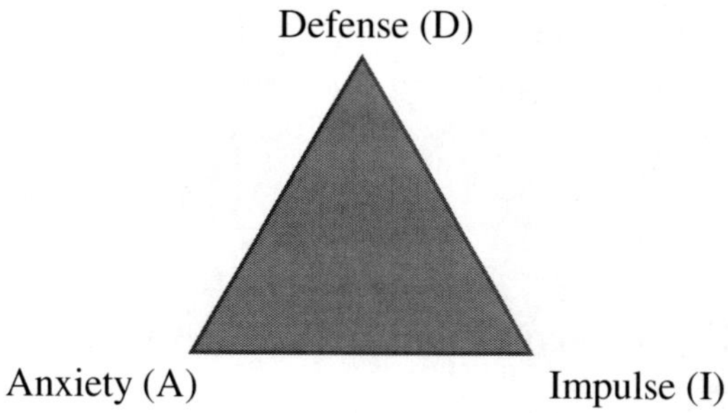

Figure 3. The Triangle of Conflict, Ezriel, 1952.

Also during the application of MUSC, the therapist is scanning the unconscious for important information regarding the Triangle of Person. This was first discussed by Menninger [40] and is summarized in Figure 4. Basically, the important individuals in operation in the therapy room are not only the patient and the therapist, who is represented as "T." In constant dynamic equilibrium are the patient's unconscious emotions towards important people in his/her current life (for example a spouse or colleague) and past life (genetic figures). The people in the patient's current life are represented with "C" and past genetic figures are represented with "P."

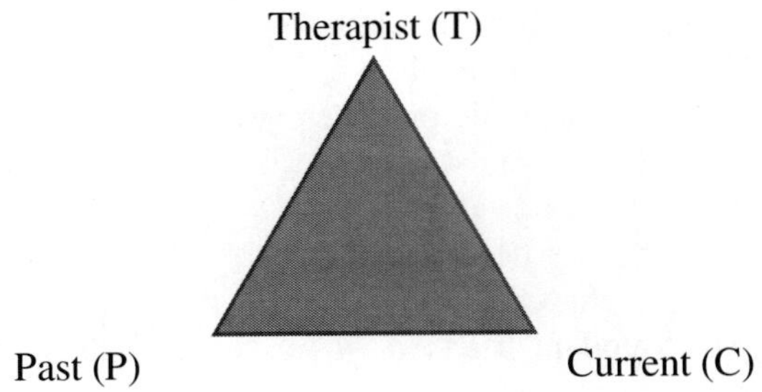

Figure 4. The Triangle of Person, Menninger, 1958.

The status of the patient's unconscious and where the unconscious is in relation to these two triangles is of paramount importance. It is the therapist's task to observe the patient, scan the unconscious, and constantly acquaint the patient with what s/he is observing.

To make this material more concrete, we will revisit the case above. During the fourth interview the patient had a breakthrough to her father. His importance in her unconscious had not been clearly appreciated before. Most of her sessions in the previous course of therapy were characterized by breakthroughs of murderous rage and guilt towards her father. After having had four sessions in the Montreal Closed Circuit Training Program, it would appear that at the pathogenic core of her unconscious are loving but conflictual relationships with both her mother and grandmother. In this light, the multiple breakthroughs towards her father in the previous treatment were not the proper zone to focus on. Most likely, the TCR was too low in that course of therapy to result in any major mobilization of her unconscious. As a result, her guilt in relation to the father was not truthfully experienced. While she does have guilt towards him, her columns of guilt towards the mother and grandmother are much greater and play a larger role in maintaining her symptom and character disturbances in life. So, at this stage, during the fourth interview in the Montreal Closed Circuit Training Program, it is important that any breakthrough she have towards the father be targeted, appropriate and reflective of his true role in the pathogenic core of her unconscious. What follows now is the vignette which occurred after she murdered the therapist and saw the visual imagery of her father.

Interviewer: How big was the knife?

Interviewee: Was there a knife? I can't remember. There was a knife in your nose.

Interviewer: What do you remember?

Interviewee: I just remember pounding.
Interviewer: What do you remember?
Interviewee: My memory was that there was a knife in your nose and I pounded. It was very powerful and I took you and pounded you in the floor.
Interviewer: What do you do with the knife?
Interviewee: What comes to mind is that it goes up the rectum. He was penetrated in life. He was a subordinate to my mother and grandmother.
Interviewer: So both of them dominated your father? Who else besides the two?
Interviewee: I added to it. I aligned with my mother and grandmother. But less so than my sisters.
Interviewer: All throughout your life?
Interviewee: Mostly since my teens.
Interviewer: Do you have a memory?
Interviewee: I had an affectionate relationship with him and then I gradually grew apart from him. We had less hugs and kisses.
Interviewer: Why are you not sure? You're not one hundred percent about being in alignment to torture your father? Why are you vague about it?
Interviewee: I didn't realize I was being vague.
Interviewer: This torture of your father and alignment with your mother and grandmother is very important. What did your father do for a living?
Interviewee: He was a fireman and then an electrician and then a fireman.
Interviewer: So his last job was a fireman. He did physical work.
Interviewee: He worked at the airport. There weren't a lot of fires. It was not that strenuous.
Interviewer: You have a memory that your mother and grandmother abused him?
Interviewee: If you consider neglect abuse, yes.
Interviewer: You have memories? How would you say his relationship is like with your mother?
Interviewee: It's very bad. I've never seen them be affectionate.
Interviewer: How was he with your mother?
Interviewee: My memory is that my mother was critical of him.
Interviewer: Could you tell me about your memory of him being scolded?
Interviewee: Once he tried to so some cleaning after he had had a few drinks. She would yell at him and be explosive. "What are you doing? Why are you using that? You've made a mess."

Interviewer: You have a specific memory? That she was openly critical that he was no good. Do you have a specific memory?
Interviewee: I do have a memory.

Employing MUSC is essential at this stage of therapy. We see that the patient is a victim of being turned against her father. Davanloo has spoken extensively of "The Syndrome of the Mother Turning the Son against the Father"[10]. These terms can be gender neutral and can refer to any configuration of a parent or grandparent turning a child against the other parent. At some point in this patient's development, she was turned against her father by her mother and grandmother. The father was subsequently deprived of loving and affectionate relationships with his four children. This highly destructive pattern is not immediately obvious to the patient, despite her mobilized unconscious. Unless these destructive forces are highlighted repeatedly, the patient will continue to be destructive. In order to change, she needs to be made aware of what needs to change. Otherwise, without this emphasis, the destructiveness will continue and be passed on to the next generation.

Highlighting these destructive forces, and the patient's role in maintaining them, is of paramount importance. While this is just a brief description of the use of MUSC in this interview, it serves to illustrate the importance of following the trail of the unconscious and using a variety of interventions to better acquaint the patient with her defensive organization and her destructiveness. Otherwise, she cannot make sense of how her unconscious maintains an active role in maintaining her current symptom and character disturbances.

CONCLUSION

This chapter has provided a review of Davanloo and his Metapsychology of the unconscious. Davanloo has not published his work since 2005 and that work has been described elsewhere. However, his most recent research findings have not previously been published in detail. This chapter serves to incorporate his newer findings by weaving in technical material and clinical vignettes from his Montreal Closed Circuit Training Program. In this light, Davanloo is not seen as a historical figure; rather his current training program is reviewed and vignettes are provided from it. Davanloo's focus on experiential, competency based psychotherapy education is unique in the field.

While some of his newer findings were reviewed, it is important to note that there are many others that were not covered. Further research is needed and findings must be disseminated to all who are interested in the field.

REFERENCES

[1] Freud S. Analysis Terminable and Interminable. Standard Edition of the Compelte Psychological Works of Sigmud Freud. 23. London: Hogarth Press; 1996. p. 209-54.

[2] Freud S. The interpretation of dreams. Standard Edition of the Complete Psychological Works of Sigmund Freud. 4. London: Hogarth Press; 1996. p. 4-5.

[3] Freud S. The Question of Lay Analysis. Standard Edition of the Complete Psychological Works of Sigmund Freud. 20. London: Hogarth Press; 1996. p. 177-250.

[4] Alexander F, French T. *Psychoanalytic Therapy: Principles and Application.* New York: Ronald Press; 1946.

[5] Malan D. Individual psychotherapy and the science of psychodynamics. New York, New York: Plenum Press.; 1979.

[6] Sifneos P. Short-Term Dynamic Psychotherapy: Evaluation and Technique: Springer; 1987.

[7] Mann J. *Time-Limited Psychotherapy.* Boston: Harvard University Press; 1980.

[8] Carlson T. A Short-Term Dynamic Psychotherapy Approach for College Students. *Journal of College Student Psychotherapy.* 2004;18(3):47-67.

[9] Bowlby J. Maternal Care and Mental Health: World Health Organization Monograph.; 1951.

[10] Davanloo H, editor. *Montreal Closed Circuit Training Program;* 2015; Montreal, Canada.

[11] APA, editor. Diagnostic and statistical manual of mental disorders. 5th ed. Washington, DC.2013.

[12] Hickey C. Davanloo's Technique of Total Removal of Resistance and Optimum Mobilization of the Transference Component of the Resistance. *Psychodynamic Psychiatry.* 2015;43(4):601-21.

[13] Davanloo H, editor. 35th Annual Metapsychology Meeting; 2014 October; Montreal, Canada.

[14] Davanloo H. *Intensive Short-Term Dynamic Psychotherapy.* Chichester, England: Wiley; 2000.

[15] Beeber A. The perpetrator of the unconscious in Davanloo's new metapsychology. Part I: Review of classic psychoanalytic concepts. *International Journal of Intensive Short-Term Dynamic Psychotherapy,* 1999;13:151-7.
[16] Davanloo H, editor. Audiovisual Immersion Course on the Metapsychological Conceptualization of Character Resistance, Transference, Guilt, and Unconscious Therapeutic Alliance in Davanloo's Psychoanalytic Technique; 1996; Bad Ragaz, Switzerland.
[17] Davanloo H, editor. Proceedings of the Fifteenth Annual European Audiovisual Symposium on Davanloo's Psychoanalytic Technique, sponsored by the Italian Institute for Intensive Short-Term Dynamic Psychotherapy and the Department of Psychiatry of the University of Florence 1997; Florence, Italy.
[18] Davanloo H, editor. Proceedings of the Sixteenth Annual European Audiovisual Symposium on Davanloo's Psychoanalytic Technique, sponsored by the German Society for Davanloo's Intensive Short-Term Dynamic Psychotherapy and the Department of Psychiatry of Friedrich-Alexander University; 1998; Erlangen, Germany.
[19] Davanloo H. Unlocking the Unconscious. Selected Papers of Habib Davanloo, MD. Chichester: Wiley; 1990.
[20] Davanloo H. Short-term dynamic psychotherapy. In: Kaplan H, Sadock B, editors. *Comprehensive Textbook of Psychiatry.* 2. 8th ed. Baltimore: Lippincott William and Wilkins; 2005.
[21] Rasmussen A, Messer S. A Comparison and Critique of Mann's Time-Limited Psychotherapy and Avalon's Short-Term Dynamic Psychotherapy. Manning Clinic, Bulletin. 2009;50(2):163-84.
[22] Parker S, Bylett M, Legett A. Challenges faced by trainee psychiatrists working towards competency in psychotherapies. *Australasian Psychiatry* 2013;21(1):56-9.
[23] Gottwick G, Sporder U, Tressel-Savelli F. Technical and Metapsychological roots of Davanloo's Intensive Short-Term Dynamic Psychotherapy: Part II: *Phase of Challenge. European Psychotherapy,* 2001;2(2):89-102.
[24] Gottwick G, Kettner-Werkmeister I, Wagner G. Technical and Metapsychological Roots of Davanloo's Intensive Short-Term Dynamic Psychotherapy: Part IV: The Entry of the Transference. *European Psychotherapy.* 2001;2(2):118-34.
[25] Gottwik G, Ostertag I, Weiss M. Technical and Metapsychological Roots of Davanloo's Intensive Short-Term Dynamic Psychotherapy: Part I:

Central Dynamic Sequence: Phase of Pressure. *European Psychotherapy* 2001;2(2):71-88.

[26] Gottwik G, Orbes I. Technical and Metapsychological Roots of Davanloo's Intensive Short-Term Dynamic Psychotherapy: Part III: Phase of Head-On Collision with the Resistance. *European Psychotherapy.* 2001;2(2):103-17.

[27] Hickey C. The Major Mobilization of the Unconscious and the Total Removal of Resistance in Davanloo's Intensive Short-term Dynamic Psychotherapy Part I: *An Introduction American Journal of Psychotherapy.* 2015;69(4):423-39.

[28] Yalom I. Prediction of improvement in group therapy. An exploratory study. *Archives of General Psychiatry.* 1967;17(2):159-68.

[29] Hickey C. Davanloo's Technique of Total Removal of Resistance and Optimal Mobilization of the Transference Component of the Resistance. *Psychodynamic Psychiatry.* 2015;43(4):601-21.

[30] Hickey C. The Management of Transference Neurosis in Davanloo's Intensive Short-term Dynamic Psychotherapy. *International Journal of Psychotherapy.* 2015;19(2):33-45.

[31] Frederickson J. Letter to Editor. *Psychodynamic Psychiatry* 2016.

[32] Mahoney D, Brock C, Diaz V, Freedy J, Thiedke C, Johnson A, et al. Balint Groups: The Nuts and Bolts of Making Better Doctors. The International Journal of Psychiatry in Medicine. 2013;45(4):401-11.

[33] Freud S. *Introductory lectures on psychoanalysis.* Strachey J, editor. New York: Norton; 1965.

[34] Reed G. The Transference Neurosis in Freud's Writings. *Journal of American Psychoanalytic Association.* 1990;38(2):423-50.

[35] Hickey C. The Major Mobilization of the Unconscious and the Total Removal of Resistance in Davanloo's Intensive Short-term Dynamic Psychotherapy Part II: Treating the Transference Neurosis. *American Journal of Psychotherapy.* 2015;69(4):441-54.

[36] Bowlby J. Forty-four juvenile thieves: Their characters and home life. *International Journal of Psychoanalysis.* 1944;25:107-27.

[37] Hickey C. Multidimensional unconscious structural changes in Davanloo's intensive short-term dynamic psychotherapy. Part I. *Archives of Psychiatry and Psychotherapy.* 2015;1:45-51.

[38] Hickey C. Multidimensional Unconscious Structrual Changes in Davanloo's Intensive Short-term Dynamic Psychotherapy--Part II. *Archives of Psychiatry and Psychotherapy.* 2015;1:53-7.

[39] Ezriel H. Notes on psychoanalytic Group therapy: II. Interpretation. *Research Psychiatry.* 1952;15:119.

[40] Menninger K. *Theory of psychoanalytic technique.* New York: Basic Books; 1958.

Biographical Sketch

Name: Catherine Hickey
Affiliation: Memorial University of Newfoundland
Education: B.Sc, MD, MMEd, FRCPC, ABPN

Address:

Geriatric Psychiatry Day Hospital
Miller Centre
100 Forest Rd
St. John's, NL, Canada
A1A 1E5
709 777 6717 (phone)
709 777 7004 (fax)
drcatherinehickey@gmail.com

Research and Professional Experience:

- Traineeship with Dr. Habib Davanloo, (2004-present).
- Psychiatrist at the Geriatric Psychiatry Day Hospital.
- Assistant Professor, Discipline of Psychiatry, Faculty of Medicine, Memorial University of Newfoundland.
- Masters in Medical Education completed at the University of Dundee (2014) with a research focus on competency based psychotherapy education.

Publications Last 3 Years:

Hickey C, McAleer S. Khallili, D. 2015. E-learning and Traditional Approaches in Psychotherapy Education: comparison. *Archives of Psychiatry and Psychotherapy* 4:48-52.

Hickey C., 2015. The Major Mobilization of the Unconscious and the Total Removal of Resistance in Davanloo's Intensive Short-term Dynamic

Psychotherapy. Part II: Treating the Transference Neurosis. *The American Journal of Psychotherapy.*

Hickey C., 2015. The Major Mobilization of the Unconscious and the Total Removal of Resistance in Davanloo's Intensive Short-term Dynamic Psychotherapy. *The American Journal of Psychotherapy.* 69(4).

Hickey C, McAleer S. Designing and Developing an Online Module: A 10 Step Approach. *Academic Psychiatry.* (Accepted for Publication).

Hickey C, McAleer S. Competence in Psychotherapy—the Role of E-Learning. *Academic Psychiatry.* (Accepted for Publication).

Hickey, C., 2015. Davanloo's Technique of Total Removal of Resistance and Optimal Mobilization of the Transference Component of the Resistance. *Psychodynamic Psychiatry.* 43(4): pp. 601-621.

Hickey, C., 2015. The Management of Transference Neurosis in Davanloo's Intensive Short-term Dynamic Psychotherapy. *International Journal of Psychotherapy.* 19 (2): 33-45.

Hickey C, McAleer S., 2015. A Needs Analysis for a Resident Psychotherapy Curriculum. *J Psychology Psychotherapy* 5:188. doi: 10.4172/2161-0487.1000188.

Hickey, C., 2015. Multi-dimensional Unconscious Structural Changes in Davanloo's Intensive Short-term Dynamic Psychotherapy: Part I. *Archives of Psychiatry and Psychotherapy* (1), pp. 45-51.

Hickey, C., 2015. Multi-dimensional Unconscious Structural Changes in Davanloo's

Intensive Short-term Dynamic Psychotherapy: Part II. *Archives of Psychiatry and Psychotherapy* (1), pp. 53-57.

Esau, D. and Hickey, C., 2013. Autonomy of Exploitation? *Hastings Center Report.* 43 (6), pp. 13-14.

In: Psychotherapy
Editor: Dominic Brewer
ISBN: 978-1-63485-226-5

Chapter 8

PRESENCE OR ABSENCE OF TRANSFERENCE NEUROSIS

***Irene Ostertag*[1], *MD*,**
and Atessa Firouz-Petermann*[2], *MA
[1]Specialist in internal medicine, psychotherapy, Nuremberg, Germany
[2]Sociologist and therapist, Geneva, Switzerland

Differential criteria in Davanloo's Intensive Short-Term Dynamic Psychotherapy used to determine the presence or absence of a Transference Neurosis based on the analysis of an interview conducted in a Closed Circuit Experiental Training Workshop setting in Montreal, Canada

ABSTRACT

In the first part of this article the authors will introduce Davanloo's Intensive Short-Term Dynamic Psychotherapy; they will present an overview of Davanloo's definition of Transference Neurosis[1] as well as his classification of 3 categories of patients:

---

[1] [...] [transference neurosis] can best be described as a situation in which the patient has transferred all of his character resistance and underlying complex neurotic feelings onto the therapist while maintaining all these neurotic forces locked up within his unconscious (Davanloo 2009).

- Patients without Transference Neurosis TN (group 1),
- Patients with the Intergenerational Destructive Competitive form of Transference Neurosis IDCTN (group 2),
- Patients with IDCTN and TN developed during psychotherapy (group 3)[2].

In the second part of the article the authors will present and analyze the technique of Major Mobilization of the Unconscious and Total Removal of the Resistance through an audiovisually recorded, transcribed interview, which took place in a Closed Circuit Experiental Training CCT Workshop[3] setting.

Our analysis of the following interview will focus on the criteria used to determine whether a TN exists or not.

The criteria are:

- The status of the Conscious and Unconscious Therapeutic Alliance UTA
- The signs of anxiety
- The kind of defense mechanisms
- The extent to which the Transference Component of the Resistance TCR increases
- The extent to which the Neurobiological Pathways NBP of rage and guilt can be activated.

In this interview we find the following parameters as indicators for the absence of a TN:

- Anxiety is present in the form of tension of the striated muscles
- Absence of malignant defenses
- Freely accessible NBPs

---

[2] The first group consists of highly resistant patients with symptom and character disturbances. There has been a fusion of primitive murderous rage and guilt dating back to the age of 4 and after; there is no TN. Patients in the second group present a complex unconscious with fusion of murderous torturous and sadistic rage, sexuality and guilt dating back to birth or the first years of life with or without TN. The third group consists of patients with an IDCTN fused with a TN developed in the course of psychotherapy or in a professional setting.

[3] A Closed Circuit Live Interview is an interview which is embedded in an experiential training workshop with the following set-up: psychotherapists trained in IS-TDP and working with the technique meet during 5-6 consecutive days to conduct interviews. In these interviews, they are in the seat of the therapist or in that of the patient alternatively. There is ongoing supervisory work by Dr. Davanloo either at the end or in between interviews.

- Sufficient rise of the TCR
- Breakthrough of primitive but not sadistic or torturous Murderous Rage as evidenced by the absence of knife, axe or other equipment

To summarize: Though the patient was highly resistant, trauma occured after age 4.

No signs of TN were elicited in the process of the interview. Taken together TN can

be ruled out in this case.

In this article, the authors use capital letters to designate Davanloo's operative concepts.

An index of the concepts and their acronym, when there is one, is to be found at the end of this article.

INTRODUCTION

The metapsychology and the technique of Intensive Short-Term Dynamic Psychotherapy IS-TDP have been developed by Habib Davanloo MD, Professor Emeritus of psychiatry at McGill University in Montreal, Canada, for over more than 50 years, based on empirical research using video technology (Davanloo 2005).

The standard technique is effective for patients suffering from phobic, obsessional, depressive and panic disorders, posttraumatic stress disorders and somatization and - with some modifications - for patients with fragile character and structural pathology.

Concentrating on emotions in the Transference, the therapist mobilizes conscious and Unconscious Therapeutic Alliance (UTA), the Transference Component of the Resistance (TCR) (Davanloo, 2014), (formerly Complex Transference Feelings) unconscious anxiety and Resistance. Dealing actively with these dynamic forces, the therapist strengthens the patient's resources.

Dr. Davanloo has developed a set of specific emotion-focused interventions in the Transference. The work seeks and requires the commitment of the patient and his collaboration through the establishment of the UTA. The UTA emerges after the resistance to emotional closeness with the therapist has been overcome.

The focus is then brought on the physical experience of emotions.

The therapist monitors the activation of the NBP related to these emotions. As the TCR rises, so does the Resistance. The Resistance expresses itself through the defensive array that has been contributing, throughout the patient's life, in keeping his avoided feelings repressed.

The therapist works on deactivating the defenses as they present themselves within the transference relationship.

The therapist's task is then to bring the patient to feel those repressed intense feelings, to direct them towards him (the therapist) and thus allow the patient to face them.

The Breakthrough into the Unconscious (Davanloo, 1990) leads to a specific traumatic experience loaded with mixed feelings (rage, guilt, grief and loving feelings) related to important figures of the past that can be, then, worked through with the therapist. This provides a direct insight into the psychopathological dynamic forces, responsible for the patient's symptoms and character disturbances, leading to a relief of the symptoms and to multidimensional structural unconscious changes in the patient.

There can be multiple repeated Breakthroughs into the Unconscious related to multiple layers of traumas at the core of the patient's neurotic suffering.

Davanloo's theorizations of Transference Neurosis, Transference as a concept and as a therapeutic tool fundamentally differ from the psychoanalytic perspective.

In the psychoanalytic treatment Transference is pivotal. The patient establishes a transference relationship with the therapist within which he unconsciously re-enacts the infantile conflict lying at the core of his neurotic suffering and psychopathology.

Theoretically, the dynamic forces having thus been uncovered and brought to the surface of the patient's psyche, within the Transference relationship, can be interpreted and worked through towards the resolution of the patient's inner conflicts.

Davanloo theorizes that "transference neurosis can best be described as a situation in which the patient has transferred all of his character resistance and underlying complex neurotic feelings onto the therapist while maintaining all these neurotic forces locked up within his unconscious. Once this state is reached, it is very difficult, if not impossible, to reach those dynamic forces responsible for the patient's neurotic suffering. The therapist becomes a figure of the patient's past, which gratifies his need, including all his destructive need, why should the patient give it up? Clearly the situation cements the neurosis rather than lifting it" (Davanloo 2009). TN builds on top of the original neurosis to protect it.

In IS-TDP treatment, TN is regarded as a twofold issue of major importance and by no means as a therapeutic tool (much less as the therapeutic tool of choice as in psychoanalytic treatment).

1. TN exists as a destructive entity against patient/therapist therapeutic alliance at the unconscious level. When transferring onto the therapist the patient re-enacts the elements of his original neurosis and, most importantly, the specific unconscious defensive organization and Resistance which will forbid the therapeutic alliance and block the way to the unconscious. The first and main hindering mechanism moving forth at that point is projective anxiety and resistance to closeness with the therapist.
2. When the presenting problem is not the original neurosis, but a transference problem derived from the original neurosis, the forces of the resistance of the guilt use TN, at an unconscious level, to protect the core neurosis. The therapist's efforts are thus misdirected towards the TN and the therapeutic process is misled.

With a TN wrapped around it, the original neurosis becomes very complex: it is sealed up and becomes invisible.

In IS-TDP the establishment of a TN is viewed as an attempt by the patient's unconscious to protect the original core neurosis in order to avoid complex feelings towards early attachment figures. These feelings are mobilized when the patient's unconscious perceives the possibility of emotional closeness with the therapist and becomes alarmed by the prospect.

The non-interpretive approach in IS-TDP involves bringing the volitional healthy part of the patient to turn against his own destructiveness by helping him become aware of the defensive barrier erected against closeness with the therapist and overcome it. This will allow the Transference TCR to rise and avoided feelings to come to the surface so that the patient can experience and work through them.

Dr. Davanloo's theorizing and conceptualization of IS-TDP is an on-going evolving process.

There are now 3 major categories of patients (whereas, previously, patients were scaled on a spectrum of neuroses).

1. The first group consists of highly resistant patients with symptom and character disturbances. Patients with multiple somatization and functional disorders, with fusion of primitive murderous rage and

guilt dating back to the age of 4 and after, for which IS-TDP is the therapy of choice. Dr. Davanloo's research results indicate that patients in this group do not develop TN.

2. The second group is the intergenerational group of psychoneurotic disorders with or without additional transference neurosis. Patients in this group present a complex unconscious structure with fusion of murderous torturous and sadistic rage, sexuality and guilt, starting at birth or in the course of the first year of life. In this group there is an IDCTN passed down through the generations. Patients in this group respond well to the removal of the Resistance but the Resistance returns shortly. They need the technique of bringing about unconscious structural and intra-psychic change. Structural change means restructuring, in the adult patient, the neurobiological pathways and unconscious defensive organization corresponding to age 0 to 1 unto the neurobiological structure and defensive organization corresponding to age 4 and after. Mobilization alone is not enough to bring about this structural change: it must be followed by psychoanalytic investigation and treatment with multiple repeated breakthroughs into the unconscious.
3. The third group consists of cases with an IDCTN (Davanloo, 2015) which has become fused with TN in the course of psychoanalytic treatment or any other form of dynamic psychotherapy or in a professional setting.

This last comprises psychiatrists and therapists whose psychopathology has become fused with their patients', their supervisor's or their own therapist's psychopathology.

In the first group of disorders dating back from age 4 and after, the unconscious is not primitive, there are no tools of aggression or lethal weapons and the Murderous Rage is not torturous or sadistic when the patient visualizes the murder of the therapist and of the genetic figure. There is also no evidence of TN, as mentioned before.

For the second and third groups, with intergenerational or other forms of transference neurosis, accessing the core neurotic structure and reaching the actual experience of the Murderous Rage within the Transference with the therapist will require much higher levels of mobilization of the TCR, of the NBP of Guilt and the actual experience of guilt, of Murderous Rage and the actual experience of rage.

On what basis are these groups defined?

- The groups are scaled according to the patient's degree of resistance and the types of defenses used.
- The types of defenses are linked to the age of trauma, before or after age 4; age 4 is not meant as a set age limit: an infant aged 2 may be at a neurobiological developmental stage of a 4 year old and a 4 year old at the stage of a child aged two. It is to be regarded as a continuum.
- Nevertheless, age 4 more or less marks a qualitative change in the child's neurobiology, the pathways having become by then completely functional.
- The stage of neurobiological development of the child when trauma begins will determine the degree of impairment of the defensive organization of his unconscious. The health or impairment of the defensive organization of the unconscious can be measured through the degree of alertness and reactivity of its defense system, ranging from quick well-targeted tactical defenses to primitive projective, malignant defenses. The earlier the trauma, the higher the degree of impairment and the more primitive the defensive organization. An impaired defensive organization of the unconscious expresses itself through a sluggish system of projective and/or malignant defenses.

In the presentation and analysis of the following interview, where one therapist sits as patient and the other as therapist, the latter uses the Technique of Vertical Mobilization of the Unconscious.

The Technique of Vertical Mobilization of the Unconscious can be described as the therapist directly and simultaneously speaking to the patient on the conscious and unconscious levels, seeking the active collaboration of the volitional Conscious and the healthy Unconscious of the patient, to overcome the resistance to emotional closeness and the defenses the patient erects between himself and the therapist in an attempt to avoid his own true feelings.

In line with Davanloo's current research about TN, the criteria we shall be concentrating on, with regard equally to patient and therapist, are those indicating the presence or absence of TN.

The Interview

This interview is embedded in the Montreal Closed Circuit Experiential Training Workshop CCT with the following set-up: psychotherapists working with IS-TDP either in private practices or in hospital settings meet during 5-6 consecutive days to conduct interviews, during which they occupy either the seat of the therapist or that of the patient.

The workshops are aimed at “cleaning” the unconscious of the therapists as well as supervising their work. The technique used here is the Technique of Vertical Mobilization of the Unconscious (Davanloo 2005) and of the NBPs of rage, guilt, grief and sexuality. There is, throughout the CCT workshops, ongoing supervisory work by Dr. Davanloo either at the end of the interviews or in between. The group members watch the live interviews and, through watching, are themselves mobilized by the process.

When the interview session is over and while it is being viewed by all the group members, including the interviewer and the interviewee, each interview undergoes extensive supervision and analysis by Dr. Davanloo.

This situation is therefore unique: a training workshop mobilizing the unconscious not only of the patient but also of the therapist and of all the other participants.

It is necessary to emphasize that the CCT is a training setting and by no means designed for therapy.

We shall here examine in what way and to what extent a TN is:

- Interfering with or allowing the establishment of the UTA between patient and therapist, thus blocking or facilitating the unlocking of the patient’s unconscious.
- Hindering or allowing the application of proper pressure by the therapist towards the mobilization and rise of the TCR aimed at bringing the patient’s resistance into the Transference in the form of defenses.

The important parameters that are being monitored throughout the interview are:

- The conscious therapeutic alliance
- The partnership between the therapist and the patient
- The signs of anxiety
- The UTA
- The extent to which the TCR rises
- The kind of defense mechanisms showing up
- The extent to which the NBPs of rage and guilt can be activated.

The Interviewer is a 56 year lady therapist thereafter referred to as Therapist (TH).

The Interviewee is a 58 year old lady therapist thereafter referred to as Patient (P).

Both are members of the CCT Group.

They were not previously acquainted, professionally or otherwise.

This is their first interview together.

To begin with, the therapist points out that this is their first meeting and that the purpose of the interview is to understand the patient's difficulties and get to the engine of her problems.

What becomes immediately clear is the patient's high level of motivation to work with the therapist.

The therapist exerts Pressure on the feelings and on the Transference Component of the Resistance TCR.

TH: How do you feel right now?

P: I am anxious. My mouth is dry.

TH: You are anxious. And how do you feel in relation with me?

P: Anxious.

TH: So you are anxious.

The therapist acknowledges the anxiety.

The patient takes a sigh.

Anxiety shows up in the tensing of the striated muscles.

TH: And what do you feel towards me besides anxiety?

The Pressure on the TCR continues.

P: Anxiety is going up.

TH: You are anxious. What else do you feel?

The therapist exerts Pressure towards the transference feelings.

The patient remains silent.

The therapist takes this as a sign of resistance against emotional closeness.

TH: You are silent. Do you allow yourself to get involved here with me?

The therapist calls on the resistance against emotional closeness. In addressing the destructive force of distancing the therapist talks to the UTA and to the Resistance; the therapeutic alliance becomes more powerful.

TH: So first let us look at what you are going to do against the distancing and the barrier? The distancing is destructive here. But if you are determined to work here with me what are you going to do against the distancing?

P: I have mental flashes of me attacking you... But I don´t feel the feeling. I don't want to let you in.

TH: So still there is a destructive need in you to hold back, to put up this barrier between us. Wherever this need is coming from… This is destructive. And we still don´t know how you feel towards me. How do you feel towards me?

The therapist applies further Pressure to feelings in the Transference. The patient answers truthfully, no sign of projective anxiety ("I don't want to let you in"). The only defense so far is anxiety defending against emotional closeness.

P: I only feel anxiety.

TH: And what else do you feel besides anxiety?

The patient takes a sigh.

Psychodiagnostically anxiety is channeled in the striated muscles, which is a sure sign that the patient's capacity to tolerate anxiety is good. This in turn means that the therapist can safely go on applying Pressure.

TH: And you took a sigh. You are anxious. What else do you feel?

P: Still I feel anxious, but some anger is building up.

TH: So let's see how you feel towards me?

The NBP of Rage is beginning to build up as, in parallel, the mobilization of the NBP of anxiety decreases.

Therefore further pressure is applied to Transference Feelings.

The therapist is looking to increase the TCR.

P: Anger is going up and down.

The patient describes the physical sensation of the movement of anger (up and down in the abdomen and thorax) but still the therapist's assessment is that the TCR is not as yet high enough and exerts further Pressure on the Transference Feelings.

So far, what can be determined with some degree of certainty is that the patient has a sound unconscious defensive system, she is not trying to avoid the therapist except for the distancing and the patient's comment "I don't want to let you in" is an indication that there is no projective anxiety.

She does not use malignant or regressive defenses such as defying the therapist or becoming weepy.

There is a good conscious therapeutic collaboration on both sides but not yet enough Unconscious Therapeutic Alliance UTA. The patient is willing to work, she answers the therapist's promptings without evasiveness, which in turn allows the therapist to exert maximum Pressure and not be lured into irrelevant directions.

TH: So still there is a destructive need in you to hold back. And we still don't know how you feel towards me. How do you feel towards me?

Further Pressure is applied to Feelings in the Transference.

P: I only feel anxiety.

TH: And what else do you feel besides anxiety?

The patient takes a sigh.

Psychodiagnostically anxiety is being channeled as tension in the striated muscles.

TH: And you took a sigh. You are anxious. What else do you feel?

P: Still I feel anxious, but some anger is building up.

TH: So let's see how you feel towards me?

Further Pressure is applied to Transference Feelings.

P: Anger is going up and down.

The patient shows with her hands an up and down movement in front of her body.

Here the therapist does a Head-on Collision HOC with the Resistance and the destructiveness of the Resistance.

TH: And still you are anxious. And still there is a barrier between us. There is a part of you that wants to work here with me. And there is another part of you that wants to distance itself from me and put a barrier between us. And then the work will be useless to you and I will be useless to you.

The therapist points out the barrier and its destructiveness.

TH: You are a capable woman. You are here to work. Now my question is this: do you really want to work with me?

The patient nods.

This intervention of reminding the patient of her abilities boosts the UTA. The therapist talks to the patient on a cognitive and emotional level, simultaneously on a conscious and unconscious level.

"Do you really want to work with me?" is a Rhetorical Question addressed to the unconscious of the patient.

TH: You are a capable woman. How old are you?

P: Uhh… How old am I? 58.

TH: You are an intelligent capable woman. You are not an anxious woman, but you are making yourself anxious.

This comment about self-inflicted anxiety brings the patient's attention to her unconscious use of anxiety as a defense.

From that moment on, the position of the patient changes and the unconscious of the patient bonds with the therapist in the UTA.

Now the defense changes into a tactical defense against anger: the patient avoids eye contact with the therapist.

P: I would like to push you.

TH: How do you really experience the anger physically?

TH: You are looking away. You are avoiding my eyes.

The therapist now labels the tactical defense.

There are no signs of regressive (e.g., no weepiness) or malignant defenses (e.g., no defiance), which is another indicator of the sound unconscious defensive structure of the patient and therefore of the absence of IDCTN in the life of the patient.

HOC with the force of the resistance

TH: Still you are anxious and controlling - a 58 years old woman who wants to work here with me. Do you want to go to this destructive system of controlling and withholding? Still you keep to this crippled position and to being the slave to the master. And you hold back this upsurge of rage towards me.

The therapist calls on the Resistance of the patient against emotional closeness which will not allow the therapist to examine the deeper feelings and impulses.

The UTA shows up in the strong emotional interaction, in the defenses (mainly tactical ones) and in the increasing striated anxiety.

TH: But how do you physically experience this anger towards me?

The therapist repeats Pressure towards the experience of anger in the Transference.

P: I can feel the anger. I can feel it in my arms.

TH: I can see this rage in your eyes. How do you experience it?

The patient shows, with a movement of the hands, that the rage is moving up from the abdomen to the chest. There is a shift from anxiety and distancing to the physical experience of anger.

The relatively short time elapsed between anxiety to anger, the ease with which the therapist acknowledges the patient's anxiety without being stopped by it, the way the therapist keeps a high level of Pressure towards the actual experience of the feelings beyond the anxiety, is an indicator of the absence of TN and of the high build-up of the conscious and UTA. The therapist is not afraid of applying Pressure towards the actual experience of anger and the patient is moving on to the actual experience of anger.

TH: If you don't minimize. How do you physically experience this rage towards me?

The therapist maintains the Pressure towards the actual experience of anger in the Transference.

P: I kick you in the stomach... I smash your head against the wall.

The anxiety has decreased allowing the mobilization of the NBP of Primitive Murderous Rage.

Here occurs the de-fusion of the Primitive Murderous Rage and the Guilt which is the central element in IS-TDP: the forces of the Resistance are the forces of the Guilt.

In the therapeutic setting, Transference Resistance can be compared to a task force of defenses set in motion by the unconscious defensive organization in an attempt to push away the therapist whose questioning threatens to bring to the surface unacceptable and guilt-laden feelings.

When structured and healthy, the unconscious defensive organization mobilizes a set of swift and efficient tactical defenses.

In the case of an impaired unconscious there are no tactical defenses to be mobilized, they don't exist, and the Resistance of the Guilt will bring forth a barrage of malignant defenses such as stubbornness, defiance, sarcasm, etc.

The technique of bringing the feelings and impulse within the Transference with the therapist by way of Pressure on the TCR is the protective safeguard, the safety net that will allow the patient to experience his repressed feelings and impulses.

The Pressure the therapist exerts on the TCR is aimed at bringing about the de-fusion of the Murderous Rage and the Guilt. This is achieved by safely bringing to the surface the unconscious murderous impulse the patient has repressed all his life towards his genetic figure, and redirecting it towards the therapist, into the safety of the Transference and the therapeutic alliance.

When de-fusion takes place, the anxiety, as the first defensive move on the part of the unconscious defensive system, decreases and disappears thus clearing the NBP for the passage of the Murderous Rage

TH: So you smash my head, go on, go on.
P: And I kick you with my leg.
TH: With which leg?
P: With the right leg.
P: I kick you on your back. Then I smash your head to the ground.

The passage of Murderous Rage continues, the image is the therapist lying on the floor.

TH: So you smash my head against the floor. Go on! If you don't control anything! Don't stop!

P: Then I keep kicking your head… Your head is destroyed. Your neck is broken. Then I keep kicking you all over the room.

The murder is weaponless, neither torturous nor sadistic. The patient uses her own limbs to murder the therapist. This indicates that the trauma in the patient's life took place when the unconscious defensive system was already structured, at around age 4 and after. This, in turn, points to an absence of IDCTN in which case trauma would have begun at birth or during the first year of life, impairing the unconscious defensive system.

The passage of heavy Murderous Rage towards the therapist continues and then the visual imagery of the therapist turns into the visual imagery of the mother.

P: There is no blood. I kick you on your back. No bone remains whole. You are loose like a puppet. And I kick and kick.

TH: You have brutally murdered me. I am now lying on the floor. And then? Look at my eyes. Keep looking to my eyes. To whom do the eyes belong?

P: They are big black eyes. It is my mother. Oh no! There are tears in her eyes, she is crying!

The patient covers her face with her hands. There is heavy sobbing. The passage of Murderous Rage is over; there is no more fusion of the murderous feelings and the guilt-laden feelings.

In this passage, two events of great importance occur:

The first one is that the NBPs correctly operate in relation to one another: after having murdered the therapist, the patient is racked with a sudden and overwhelming upsurge of Guilt. The mobilizer of the Guilt is the visual imagery of the mother. The actual physical experience of the Murderous Rage clears the NBP for the subsequent passage of Guilt. And before that, the passage of Murderous Rage becomes possible when the NBP of anxiety had been cleared for the subsequent passage of Murderous Rage.

The second important event is that the NBP of Guilt is activated through the channel of the eyes. The eye contact with the visual imagery of the murdered therapist activates the transition to the visual imagery of the genetic figure and some movement in the eyes of the murdered body clearly increases the Guilt, in this case the patient sees tears in her mother's eyes.

TH: It is your mother! Don't stop, don´t stop. You have a lot of painful feelings.

P: (Loud sobbing)

TH: Let the feelings come. There is another wave of feeling.

P: They are big black eyes. It is my mother.

TH: Look at the eyes of mother, you have another painful wave. Don't fight your feelings. You owe it to yourself.

P: (Heavy waves of sobbing)

TH: Perhaps it is good to get closer to mother, don´t be distant.

The heavy extensive passage of guilt-laden feelings continues.

P: I am stroking her black hair... I should have done that long ago... I needed her so badly.

Continuation of grief and guilt-laden feelings and sadness about all that has been missed in the past.

P: I would tell her, I love her.

TH: How would you say that?

P: Mummy, I love you so much.

There are more painful waves of feelings.

P: I am so sorry. I want to be close. No, actually I want to be a child again; I want to be in her arms. It is too late now, she is dead, and it is all gone.

The process enters the phase of analysis and recapitulation. The patient has seen the image of her mother at the age of approximately 40, which was 46 years ago when she, herself, was 11-12 years old. The patient is not able at that moment to calculate correctly. Memories come back about having missed her so much.

P: I needed her so badly and I didn't want to feel the need …When I was sent to boarding school, at around the age of 5-6, I needed her and she wasn't there for me. So from then on I never let her close to me again. I didn't want to feel the need of her.

During this phase there are, again, passages of Guilt and loving feelings.

Then the session is brought to closure. It lasted 25 minutes.

As mentioned before, the establishment of trauma at age of 5-6 is important in that it shows the type of neurosis the patient has developed: no TN, no malignant defenses, no projective anxiety, willingness to work and a great fear of emotional closeness with anxiety as the main defense against emotional closeness.

We are dealing here with the original neurosis.

Also as mentioned before, the weaponless murder points to the fact that trauma took place after the age of 4: she uses her body strength, hands, arms, feet, legs, to murder the therapist.

One could hypothesize that this shows the state of the patient's body strength and development of the NBPs at the age the trauma happened.

The visual imagery could be tapping into the stream of a child's unconscious aged 5-6, who is, at that point, strong and powerful enough to feel she can murder without enhancing her strength with lethal weapons.

CONCLUSION

The interview lasted around 25 minutes.

It started with the phase of Pressure: Pressure towards the experience of feelings in the Transference and Pressure to the Resistance especially the resistance against emotional closeness. Then there were Head-on Collisions HOC with the Transference Resistance, the therapist directly addressing the resistance and pointing out how this resistance is a destroyer of relationships, leading to a rise in the TCR and to the mobilization of the UTA.

During this phase there has been no interpretation or analysis whatsoever. With the total removal of the resistance the patient has been able to experience the NBPs of the Primitive Murderous Rage, which is in relation to her mother and dates back to almost 50 years, followed by guilt and grief and loving feelings.

There was a Total Removal of the Resistance, leading to a major Breakthrough. The analysis showed the biographical background.

As we have seen, the parameters which are indicators for the absence of TN in the patient under these special circumstances can be summarized as follows:

- Anxiety shows in the form of striated anxiety, tension of the striated muscles.
- There are no signs for malignant defenses.
- The NBPs are freely accessible.
- The TCR can develop.
- The Breakthrough is primitive but not sadistic or torturous, there is no use of knife or axe or other lethal equipment.

ACKNOWLEDGMENTS

In this article the authors have used a set of concepts and technical interventions such as Pressure, Breakthrough (previously Unlocking of the Unconscious), Transference Component of the Resistance TCR (previously Complex Transference Feelings), Unconscious Therapeutic Alliance UTA, and Neurobiological Pathways of Rage and Guilt (NBPs of R and G), Head-on Collision (HOC). All of these concepts and interventions come from Dr. Davanloo's published and unpublished work.

Additionally the authors have made references to metapsychological conceptualizations from Dr. Davanloo's live teachings.

We want to thank Dr. Davanloo for his teaching and intensive supervisory work.

INDEX OF KEY CONCEPTS AND ANCRONYMS

- Breakthrough into the Unconscious (formerly Unlocking the Unconscious)
- CCT Closed Circuit Experiential Training Workshop
- De-fusion of the Murderous Rage and the Guilt
- Transference Feeling, Feelings in the Transference
- Guilt
- HOC Head-on Collision with the Resistance

- IDCTN Intergenerational Destructive Competitive form of Transference Neurosis
- IS-TDP Davanloo´s Intensive Short-Term Dynamic Psychotherapy
- Major Mobilization of the Unconscious
- Neurobiological Pathways
- Primitive Murderous Rage, Murderous Rage
- R Resistance
- Resistance against emotional closeness
- Resistance of the Guilt
- Rhetorical Question
- TCR Transference Component of the Resistance (formerly Complex Transference Feelings)
- Total Removal of the Resistance
- TN Transference Neurosis
- T Transference
- Transference Resistance, Resistance
- UTA Unconscious Therapeutic Alliance
- Vertical Mobilization of the Unconscious

REFERENCES

Davanloo, H. (1990). *Unlocking the Unconscious: Selected Papers of Habib Davanloo, M.D.*, Chichester: Wiley.

Davanloo, H. (2005). Intensive Short-Term Dynamic Psychotherapy. In: H. Kaplan and B. Sadock (Eds.), *Comprehensive Textbook of Psychiatry* (8th ed., Vol. II). Baltimore: Lippincott Williams and Wilkins.

Davanloo, H. (2009). *Collected Papers of H. Davanloo, M.D.*, Transference Neurosis: clinical, technical, metapsychological and ethical considerations, March 2009.

Davanloo, H. (2014). *Collected Papers of H. Davanloo, M.D.*, The Technique of Total Removal of Resistance, June 2014.

Davanloo, H. (2015). *Collected Papers of H. Davanloo, M.D.*, Intergenerational Transference Neurosis, January 2015.

Curriculum vitae

Dr. med Irene Margarete Ostertag
Fachärztin für Innere Medizin, Psychotherapie
Fürther Str. 62
90429 Nürnberg
Tel. 0049(0)911267400

1958 Born in Heidelberg
1964-1977 School Education in Heidelberg and Ulm
1977-1984 Medical School in Ulm, Tübigen and Vienna
1984 M.D. and License to Practice Medicine
1984-1985 Assistant at the Department of Oncology at the University of Ulm
1985-1993 Assistant and Senior Physician at the Municipal Hospital of Nuremberg, continuus education in Internal Medicine with a specialization in oncology
1993 Exam as specialist in Internal Medicine
1989-1993 Continuous training in Psychodynamic Psychotherapy at the Institute of Psychotherapy (Nürnberger Weiterbildungskreis für Psychotherapie) affiliated to the clinic of Psychosomatic Medicine and Psychotherapy of the Municipal Hospital of Nuremberg
Since 1993 Registerd Doctor and Practitioner for General Medicine, Internal Medicine and Psychotherapy in Nuremberg
Since 1996 Member of the German Society of Davanloo's Intensive Short-term Dynamic Psychotherapy
Since 1996 Training with Dr. Davanloo in Switzerland, Germany and Canada
Since 2006 Supervisor and teacher in Psychodynamic Psychotherapy
Since 2007 Instructor of IS-TDP Training Program in Nuremberg
Since 2012 Participation in Workshops with supervision by Dr. Davanloo in Montreal
Since 2012 Leader of Balint Groups by approval of the German Balint Federation and of the Medical Association of the State of Bavaria
Since 2015 President of the German Society of Davanloo's Internsive Short-term Dynamic Psychotherapy

Curriculum vitae

Atessa, Firouz Petermann
President of D-ISTDP Swiss Institute for H. Davanloo's Technique of Total Removal of the Resistance, Major Mobilization of the Unconscious and ISTDP

E-mail: atessafirouz@yahoo.fr

Date of birth: March 5th 1956
Place of birth: Rome, Italy
Nationality: Swiss and Iranian
Marital status: Married, two children (1988 and 1990)

Professional address
CCPP Cabinet Consultation Psychologie and Psychothérapie
8, Place de Grenus
CH-1201 Geneva, Switzerland
Prof. Phone: +41 22 731 72 73

Home address
5, Chemin des Lucioles
CH-1234 Vessy, Switzerland
Private phone: + 41 22 784 21 79
Cell phone: +41 76 379 77 63

Schooling and university
1982-1988
University of Geneva, Switzerland
1974-1975
University of Florida, Gainesville, Fla. US
1962-1973
Boarding school, primary and secondary: Collège Beau-Soleil CH-1884 Villars-sur-Ollon
(Vaud) Switzerland

Diplomas and degrees
2004 Physical Trainer diploma FISAF International

2001 Squash Instructor diploma with Jeunesse et Sports Suisse Squash, OFSPO Swiss

Federal Office for Sports

2001 Master Specialist's degree in Sophrologie Caycédienne, social prophylaxis section

and sports section, Geneva, Switzerland and Principality of Andorra with Dr. Psych.

Alfonso Caycedo

1988 Master's degree in Sociology, University of Geneva, Switzerland

1973 French baccalaureat option philosophy

Current studies and continuing education

2014-on CCT Closed Circuit Training with Dr. Psych. H.Davanloo Montreal, Canada

Supervisors in Switzerland: Dr. Psych. M. Fournier and Dr. Psych. R. Bandettini

2014 ASTRAG Association pour le travail Groupal thérapeutique et social – Association

for socially therapeutical group work with Dr. psych. G. Galli-Carminati, Geneva,

Switzerland.

2013-on ISTDP Intensive Short-Term Dynamic Psychotherapy studies

Professional experience

In the field of therapeutic work

Working languages: French, English, Persian, Dari Afghani

2015-on President for D-ISTDP Swiss Institute for H. Davanloo's Technique of Total

Removal of the Resistance, Major Mobilization of the Unconscious and ISTDP

2012-on Geneva, Switzerland

Private practice: 8, Place de grenus, CH-1201 GE

ISTDP Intensive Short-term Dynamic Psychotherapy (supervised)

Supportive therapy

Sophrology

Sophrology sports mental training

Analytical individual psychodrama in group setting and individually
EMDR Eye Movement Desensitization and Reprocessing
Volunteer therapeutical work with Asylum seekers in Switzerland

2008-2010 Téhéran, Iran
Private practice of Dr. M-V Sahami, Child psychiatrist DPM, MRCPsych, DM
Supportive therapy, Individual psychodrama, sophrology
Work with traumas associated with war conditions, forced migration issues associated
with war, rural-urban adjustment problems, acculturation process issues, moral violence
and marital violence, work with women
Analytical individual psychodrama

2001-2008 Geneva, Switzerland
Private practice: 10, Place de Grenus, 1201, Genève
Supportive therapay
Sophrology
Sophrology sports mental training
Individual analytical psychodrama
EMDR Eye Movement Desensitization and Reprocessing

In the field of translation and interpretation
French, English, Persian, Dari afghani
2012-on
Administrative Detention Center LMC Frambois, Geneva: for psychologist, psychiatrist,
medical staff, social worker and administrative staff

Police and law enforcement authorities – Office of the State Counsel – Labour courts
In cantons Geneva, Vaud and Fribourg, Switzerland

In the field of volunteer work
2011-2013
Legal representative for the Association ELISA.ASILE, 2 rue de la Roseraie, 1205
Geneva, Switzerland

Free Legal assistance, interpretation-translation and social assistance for asylum seekers

In the field of sports

2008-2009 Iran

Private coaching in Squash, Revolution Sports Club

2001-2006 Suisse

Squash Instructor Bois-Carré Sports Club and Cologny Sports Club, Geneva

Team trainer and captain for the Chambésy Squash Club Women's teams, Geneva

Mental training for the Bossey Golf Club Women's team, France

Index

A

B

C

D

E

F

G

H

I

O

P

T

U

W